The Best 100 Keto Diet Recipes

Esther J. Keller

Table of Contents

Breakfast Recipes

Coco Pancakes

Ingredients

- Almond flour ½ cup
- Flax seed meal ½ cup
- Eggs 4
- Raw honey 2 tbsp.
- Almond oil 4 tsp.
- Coconut milk ½ cup
- Erythritol 4 tsp.
- Ghee 2 tbsp.
- Coconut flour 1 tsp.
- Baking powder 1 tsp.
- Nutmeg ¼ tsp.
- Cinnamon ½ tsp.
- Pinch salt

Preparation Method

- First, mix the almond flour, flax seeds, erythritol, salt and baking powder together in bowl.
- Mix all the dry ingredients together well so everything is distributed evenly; add eggs to the mixture and mix well.
- Mix until a liquid consistency is achieved and add almond oil, honey and milk together. Mix again to a liquid consistency.
- Add coconut flour, spices to mixture and mix well.

- In a skillet, heat ghee and coconut oil and add 1/4 cup of pancake mix
- Cook until brown color and remove from pan. Before serving, add a little maple syrup and enjoy the taste!

Nutritional Information

- Preparation Time: 20 minutes
- Total servings: 8
- Calories: 222.5 (per serving)
- Fat: 22.4g
- Protein: 6.5g
- Carbs: 1.7g

Walnut Crush with Cauliflower

Ingredients

- Walnuts 7/8 cup (crushed)
- Flax seeds 2 oz
- Chia seeds 2 oz
- Cauliflower 2 oz (Riced)
- Coconut milk 3 cups
- Cream ¼ cup
- Cream cheese 2 oz
- Butter 1 tbsp.
- Ghee 2 tbsp.
- Protein powder 2 tbsp.
- Cinnamon 1 tsp.
- Maple flavor 1 tsp.
- Vanilla extract ½ tsp.
- Nutmeg ¼ tsp.
- Allspice ¼ tsp.
- Erythritol 1 oz

Preparation Method

- Mix flax and chia seeds in small cup and put aside. In a food processor, add riced cauliflower, protein powder and keep aside.
- Toast the raw walnuts in pan (before you toast, smash walnuts into small pieces)

- In another pan, add coconut milk and boil until it's cooked well.
- Decrease heat under pan and add cinnamon, maple, vanilla, nutmeg and allspice. Add erythritol and stir well.
- Now, add flax seeds and chia seeds to the pan and mix well. When it starts to thicken tremendously.
- Add cream, butter, ghee, walnuts, and mix together well and make it a bit thicker and enjoy the taste!

Nutritional Information

- Preparation Time: 15 minutes
- Total servings: 6
- Calories: 466.6 (per serving)
- Fat: 33.7g
- Protein: 12.4g
- Carbs: 4.4g

Creamy Smashed Egg

Ingredients

- Bacon fat 1 tbsp
- Large Eggs 2
- Ghee 1 tbsp
- Cheddar cheese 2 tbsp
- Cilantro 1 tbsp.
- Salt and pepper to taste

Preparation Method

- Before heating pan, shred the cheese and chop the cilantro.
- Now heat the pan with bacon fat on medium low heat, add eggs, cilantro, salt and pepper.
- Once the edges start to turn to a light brown color, add ghee on top and start smashing until it becomes small pieces.
- Switch off pan and add cheese in the center and start mixing from four sides.
- Cook until it turns to a slightly golden color and if desired, enjoy with cooked bacon slices!

Nutritional Information

- Preparation Time: 15 minutes
- Total servings: 1
- Calories: 222
- Fat: 31.3g
- Protein: 16.1g

- Carbs: 2.3g

Honey Pancakes

Ingredients

- Coconut meal 1 cup
- Large eggs 2
- Honey 1 tbsp.
- Pumpkin puree 2 fl oz
- Cream ¼ cup
- Ghee 1 tbsp.
- Butter 1 tbsp.
- Pumpkin pie spice 1 tsp
- Baking powder ½ tsp
- Salt to taste

Preparation Method

- Mix eggs, pumpkin puree, honey, cream and ghee together without lumps.
- Mix coconut meal, pumpkin pie spice, baking powder and salt together in a separate bowl.
- Slowly start adding the wet mixture (Step 1) to get a smooth consistency by adding butter.
- Heat the pan and grease the pan with butter, then add the pancake batter into the pan and cook until bubbles appear on the top.
- Flip it and cook the other side until browned and serve it warm for a nice taste!

Nutritional Information

- Preparation Time: 15 minutes
- Total servings: 8
- Calories: 191.5 (per serving)
- Fat: 15.7g
- Protein: 5.8g
- Carbs: 2g

Bacon Butter Eggs

Ingredients
- Bacon 4 slices
- Large eggs 5
- Rinds 2 oz
- Tomato 1
- Avocado 1
- Butter 1 tbsp.
- Green pepper 2
- White onion 1 oz
- Watercress 2 tbsp.
- Salt and pepper to taste

Preparation Method
- Dice all vegetables listed above.
- Fry meat in a pan with butter and in another pan fry rinds.
- Once the rinds are crispy, add vegetables to the pan and mix them together until they are mixed well; seasoned as needed.
- Once onions are translucent, add chopped watercress to the pan, mix everything together, add bacon and allow it to cook for 2 minutes.
- Add eggs and mix everything together and let it cook like an omelet.

- Before serving, add avocado cubes and mix. Enjoy the delicious taste!

Nutritional Information

- Preparation Time: 25 minutes
- Total servings: 3
- Calories: 539.8 (per serving)
- Fat: 44.8g
- Protein: 24.2g
- Carbs: 5.1g

Cheese Omelet

Ingredients
- Bacon 2 slices (cooked)
- Bacon fat 1 tbsp.
- Chopped orange pepper 2 tbsp.
- Large eggs 2
- Ghee 1 tbsp
- Cheddar cheese 2 tbsp
- Chives 2 stalks
- Salt and pepper to taste

Preparation Method
- Before heating pan, shred the cheese and cooked bacon and chop the chives.
- Now heat the pan with bacon fat on medium low heat, add eggs, chives, salt and chopped orange pepper.
- Once the edges start to turn a light brown color, add bacon to the center of the pan and cook for 30 seconds by adding ghee on top.
- Switch off pan and add cheese to the center and start folding from four sides of omelet slowly.
- Now, turn the omelet and cook them until it turns to a slightly golden color. Enjoy the delicious bacon omelet!

Nutritional Information

- Preparation Time: 15 minutes
- Total servings: 1
- Calories: 599
- Fat: 52.1g
- Protein: 24.6g
- Carbs: 4.4g

Maple Waffles

Ingredients

Waffles:

- Almond flour ½ cup
- Flax seeds 1 ½ tbsp.
- Coconut milk 1/3 cup
- Vanilla extract ½ tsp.
- Baking powder 1 tsp.
- Eggs 2
- Swerve 1 ½ tbsp
- Butter 1 tbsp
- Liquid stevia 10 drops

Filling:

- Maple syrup 1/3 cup
- Half orange zest
- Orange juice 2 tsp.
- Ghee 1 tbsp.
- Swerve 1 tbsp.
- Brie cream 1/3 cup

Preparation Method

- Mix all the ingredients for the waffles in a container and mix until it looks smooth.

- Add your batter to the waffle maker or small pan and after cooking to allow them to cool.
- Slice your brie and lay on top of your waffles while still warm. In a pan, heat both the ghee and swerve on medium heat until it brown. Then add honey, orange juice, and orange zest.
- Continue to stir the mixture until it bubbles and becomes like jam. On the other side, heat the waffle until brie starts melting.
- Now, add filling and brie together and put on the pan and grill for 1-2 per side; enjoy the taste with a little honey on top!

Nutritional Information

- Preparation Time: 20 minutes
- Total servings: 12
- Calories: 520 (2 pieces per serving)
- Fat: 41.8g
- Protein: 21g
- Carbs: 7.3g

Quick Sausage Casserole

Ingredients

- Sausage 1 lb (beef)
- Zucchini 0.5 lb
- Cabbage 0.5 lb
- Onion 1.5 oz
- Large eggs 3
- Ghee 1 tbsp.
- Butter 1 tbsp.
- Mayonnaise ½ cup
- Mustard seeds 1 ½ tsp.
- Ground sage 1 tsp.
- Cheddar cheese 6 oz
- Red pepper flakes to taste

Preparation Method

- Preheat the oven to 375F and grease a casserole dish with ghee and keep aside.
- In a large skillet, cook the sausage on a medium heat for 10 minutes.
- Add cabbage, zucchini, and onion and cook until vegetables are tender and sausage is fully cooked.
- In a separate bowl, mix eggs, mayonnaise, mustard, sage and pepper until smooth. Add grated cheese to egg mixture and stir.

- Add this mixture to the casserole dish and top it with little extra cheese. Bake for 30 minutes in a preheated oven or until bubbling around the edges.
- After 30 minutes, remove from oven, add 1 tbsp. of butter and serve immediately.

Nutritional Information

- Preparation Time: 40 minutes
- Total servings: 6
- Calories: 524.6 (per serving)
- Fat: 44.9g
- Protein: 19.3g
- Carbs: 4.8g

Almond Cupcakes

Ingredients

- Almond flour 500g
- Cocoa powder 60g
- Protein powder 45g
- Baking soda 10g
- Xanthan gum 2g
- Salt 2g
- Purified butter 70g
- Swerve sweetener 50g
- Large eggs 2
- Root beer extract 10g
- Stevia extracts 2g
- Glaze:
- Whipped cream 240g
- Powdered Swerve sweetener 55g
- Vanilla extract 2g

Preparation Method

- For cakes, preheat the oven to 325F and use muffin pan with paper feed (or use the stand-alone liner).
- In a medium-sized bowl, add almond flour, cocoa powder, protein, baking powder, xanthan gum, salt and mix well.
- In a large bowl, beat butter with erythritol until creamy. Mix eggs, then beat in root berry extract and stevia extract.

- Beat in almond blend in two batches, alternating with sugar-free root beer and scraping off sides of bowl and bats as needed. Divide dough between prepared muffins. Bake 25 minutes.
- Allow to cool in the pan. For the icing on the cake, combine cream, powdered erythritol and vanilla extract in large bowl. Beat until stiff peaks form but do not surpass. Pipe or spoon on chilled cupcakes.

Nutritional Information

- Preparation Time: 35 minutes
- Total servings: 12
- Calories: 267 (per serving)
- Fat: 25 g
- Protein: 10g
- Carbs: 4g

Butter Cheesecake

Ingredients

- Butter 115g
- Unsweetened chocolate 55g
- Almond flour 120g
- Cocoa powder 60g
- Salt to taste
- Large eggs 2
- Sweetener 50g
- Vanilla 2g
- Walnuts 30g
- Fresh cheese 450g
- Large eggs 2
- Swerve sweetener 100g
- Heavy cream 60g
- Vanilla extract 2g

Preparation Method

- For the brownie base, preheat the oven to 325F and butter a 9-inch pan. Wrap bottom of the pan with foil. In a microwaveable bowl or glass measuring cup, melt butter and chocolate together in the microwave for 30 seconds.
- In a small bowl, beat almond flour, cocoa powder and salt. In a large bowl, beat eggs, swerve and vanilla until smooth.

Beat in almond flour mixture, then butter chocolate mixture until smooth. Stir in the nuts.

- Spread evenly over the bottom of the prepared pan. Bake 20 minutes, until around the edges, but still soft in the middle. Leave to cool for 15 minutes.
- For the filling, reduce the oven temperature to 300F. In a large bowl, beat the fresh cheese until smooth. Beat in eggs, swerve, cream and vanilla until well combined.
- Pour filling over crust and square cheesecake on a large biscuit sheet. Bake until the edges are set and the center wiggles only slightly (45 minutes). Remove from the oven and allow cooling.
- Run a knife to release the edges and then remove the sides of the pan. Cover with plastic film and store in a refrigerator for at least 3 hours. Serve with sugar-free chocolate sauce.

Nutritional Information

- Preparation Time: 80 minutes
- Total servings: 10
- Calories: 381 (per serving)
- Fat: 33g
- Protein: 8.68g
- Carbs: 4.2g

Nut Bread

Ingredients

- Eggs 6
- Sour cream 170g
- Baking soda 2g
- Garlic powder 2g
- Onion powder 2g
- Salt 2g
- Protein powder 60g
- Brazil nuts 56g
- Mascarpone 56g
- Heavy cream 110g

Preparation Method

- Preheat oven at 300F. Place your egg white, cream in a blender until stiff and put aside.
- Put the egg yolks with the remaining ingredients in a bowl and mix well. Fold in a small amount of egg whites into the yolk mixture a little at a time.
- Pour them into a greased loaf pan and add smashed brazil nuts as a topping. Bake for 60 minutes (to test, use a toothpick to see if it goes in and comes out of the middle cleanly)
- Allow to cool before removing and cutting. Keep refrigerated.

Nutritional Information

- Preparation Time: 75 minutes
- Total servings: 12
- Calories: 115 (per serving)
- Fat: 14.3g
- Protein: 8.3g
- Carbs: 1.33g

Pumpkin Cheese Bread

Ingredients

Bread:

- Almond flour 7 oz.
- Pumpkin pie spice mix 2 tsp.
- Cream of tartar 1 tsp.
- Baking soda 1/4 tsp.
- Orange zest 1 tbsp
- Ghee 2 oz
- Eggs 4
- Erythritol 3 oz.
- Cinnamon 1 tsp.
- Pumpkins puree 5 oz.

Topping:

- Cream cheese 21 oz.
- Egg 1
- Orange juice 1.5 fl oz.
- Erythritol 1.5 oz.
- Stevia extract 10 drops
- Cinnamon ½ tsp.
- Pumpkins puree 3.5 oz.
- Orange zest 1 tbsp.
- Pinch of salt

Preparation Method

- At first, preheat the oven to 300F. In a large bowl, add almond flour, cinnamon, pumpkin pie spice, cream of tartar, baking soda and mix well.
- Add eggs, ghee, erythritol, cinnamon and mix well.
- Add a spoon of pumpkin puree and mix well (fresh pumpkin puree gives a better taste then canned puree).
- Now, add juice and zest (half of an orange) and mix. In another bowl, prepare the cheesecake topping by mixing all topping ingredients.
- Spoon the bread batter into a baking dish suitable for bread and distribute evenly using a ladle. Add a layer using half of the cheese mixture on top of the bread batter and spread evenly.
- Mix the remaining cheese mixture with the pumpkin puree. Gently spoon the pumpkin cheese mixture on top and spread evenly. Transfer into the preheated oven and bake for 60 minutes, make sure that bread is not going too burnt on top.
- Carefully remove from the baking dish, slice into 12 pieces and enjoy the taste.

Nutritional Information

- Preparation Time: 80 minutes
- Total servings: 12
- Calories: 300 (per serving)
- Fat: 29.33g
- Protein: 10g
- Carbs: 5.5g

Cranberry Muffins

Ingredients

- Almond flour ½ cup
- Flax seed meal ½ cup
- Eggs 4
- Raw honey 2 tbsp.
- Almond oil 4 tsp.
- Coconut milk ½ cup
- Erythritol 4 tsp.
- Ghee 2 tbsp.
- Coconut flour 1 tsp.
- Baking powder 1 tsp.
- Nutmeg ¼ tsp.
- Cinnamon ½ tsp.
- Pinch salt

Preparation Method

- At first, preheat your oven to 350F. In a bowl, add egg yolks, ghee, stevia and swerve. Mix until creame paste.
- Now, add the orange zest, almond, coconut flour, Chia seeds, cinnamon, baking soda, pinch salt and combine well. Pour in the coconut milk and mix until combined well.
- Meantime, whip the egg whites with the cream of tartar until they create soft peaks. Gently add them into the dough and mix completely.

- Halve the cranberries and add them to the dough. Grease the muffin cups with ghee to avoid sticking and add batter into muffin cups.
- Place these muffin cups in preheated oven for 30 minutes until the tops turn to golden brown. When it finishes, let it cool for 10 minutes and enjoy the taste.

Nutritional Information

- Preparation Time: 40 minutes
- Total servings: 10
- Calories: 225.8 (per serving)
- Fat: 19.4g
- Protein: 9.3g
- Carbs: 4g

Raspberry Cream Pancakes

Ingredients

Pancakes

- Eggs 2
- Coconut flour 1 tbsp.
- Dried coconut 2 tbsp.
- Baking soda 1/4 tsp.
- Coconut milk 3 tbsp.
- Vanilla beans extract ½ tsp.
- Ghee 1 tbsp.
- Liquid Stevia 5 drops

Pancakes

- Coconut cream 4.4 oz.
- 1 vanilla bean
- Fresh raspberries 1.5 oz.
- Dried coconut 1 tsp.

Preparation Method

- At first, whisk the eggs in a small bowl and keep aside.
- In a separate bowl, mix coconut flour, dry coconut, vanilla bean extract, baking soda and mix well. Now, add egg mixture to the bowl with stevia and combine well.
- In a small bowl, mix the yogurt with vanilla bean. Wash and dice the raspberries and keep aside.

- Prepare the pan by greasing with ghee and when ghee is hot, add pancake batter and cook each side 1 minute.
- After making all pancakes, place on a serving plate and make layers of pancakes, yogurt and raspberries. Sprinkle the top with some dry coconut or fresh coconut and enjoy the taste.

Nutritional Information

- Preparation Time: 20 minutes
- Total servings: 3
- Calories: 585 (per serving)
- Fat: 42.5g
- Protein: 29g
- Carbs: 11g

Bacon Stuffed Pancakes

Ingredients

Pancake

- Thinly bacon slices 8
- Coconut flour 2 oz.
- Almond flour 6 oz.
- Protein 1 tbsp.
- Swerve 2 oz.
- Baking soda 1/2 tsp.
- Cream of tartar 1 tsp.
- Eggs 4
- Ghee 2 fl oz.
- Almond milk 16 fl oz.
- Liquid stevia 10 drops

Chocolate dip

- Cocoa powder 2 tbsp.
- Ghee 2 tbsp.
- Swerve 2 tbsp.

Preparation Method

- At first, prepare the crispy bacon by placing in oven (375F) for 15 minutes, until the bacon is browned.
- For making pancakes, combine all pancakes ingredients into a bowl and mix well.

- Heat a large pan by adding with ghee, when ghee is hot, pour the batter with regular spoon and top with slice of crispy bacon and cook for 10 minutes each side.
- Meanwhile, make chocolate dip, mix all ingredients and serve with the pancakes.

Nutritional Information

- Preparation Time: 30 minutes
- Total servings: 2 (4 pancakes per serving)
- Calories: 564 (per serving)
- Fat: 51g
- Protein: 21.3g
- Carbs: 5g

Lunch Recipes

Express Pizza

Ingredients

- Shredded mozzarella 2.4 oz.
- Shredded mascarpone 1 oz.
- Marinara sauce 4 oz.
- Pepperoni 4 slices
- Basil 1/2 tsp.
- Oregano 1/2 tsp

Preparation Method

- At first, put frying pan over medium heat and add mozzarella cheese, mascarpone cheese (keep little both cheese for topping) and cook for 5 minutes or until cheese is caramelized.
- Don't forget to use a spatula to avoid sticking it to the pan. Now, pour marinara sauce over top and spread it all over cheese.
- Sprinkle the remaining cheese's over top of that and add slices of pepperoni.
- Season with herbs (basil, oregano) and wait until the top layer of cheese has melted, let it cool for 2 minutes and enjoy the taste.

Nutritional Information

- Preparation Time: 12 minutes

- Total servings: 1
- Calories: 530 (per serving)
- Fat: 42g
- Protein: 26g
- Carbs: 8g

Apple Pork Fry

Ingredients

Pork Chops

- Pork chops 4
- Ghee 2 tbsp.
- Salt and pepper to taste
- Paprika 1 tsp.
- Small apple 1
- Rosemary 1 tsp.

Vinaigrette

- Apple cider vinegar 2 tbsp.
- Lemon juice 1 tbsp.
- Maple syrup 1 tbsp.
- Salt and pepper to taste
- Olive oil 2 tbsp.

Preparation Method

- At first, season pork chops with salt, pepper, ghee and keep aside.
- Place large iron skillet over high heat and add seasoned pork chops and cook 5 minutes each side.
- Decrease the heat to medium and add apple slices, rosemary over the pork chops and place in the oven for about 10 minutes at 350F.

- Meanwhile, prepare vinaigrette by mixing all the ingredients together.
- When pork chops are ready, pour vinaigrette over top and serve hot.

Nutritional Information

- Preparation Time: 25 minutes
- Total servings: 2
- Calories: 485 (per serving)
- Fat: 41g
- Protein: 25g
- Carbs: 4g

Chees Stuffed Cabbage

Ingredients

Batter

- Ghee 1 tbsp.
- Egg 1
- Cream cheese 1 tbsp.
- Mozzarella 1 tbsp.
- Almond flour 2 tbsp.
- Flax meal 1 tbsp.
- Baking powder 1/2 tsp.
- Salt to taste

Filling

- Shredded green cabbage 3 oz.
- Bacon slices 2

Toppings

- Mayonnaise 2 tbsp.
- Rice vinegar 1 tsp.
- BBQ sauce 1 tbsp.
- Seaweed flakes 1 tbsp.
- Bonito flakes 1 tbsp.

Preparation Method

- In a small bowl mix mayonnaise, rice vinegar and keep aside.
- In a mixing bowl, add ghee, cream cheese, mozzarella and mix until softened.
- Now, add almond flour, flax meal, baking powder, salt to the mixing bowl and mix well.
- Now, add egg into the batter, add green cabbage and stir until fully incorporated
- Place large skillet over medium heat and add sliced bacon until it becomes crispy
- Spread incorporated batter into bacon skillet and cook for 5 minutes or until batter turns to golden color on the bottom.
- Flip and cook again 5 minutes and transfer to a plate. Spread BBQ sauce, mayonnaise. Finally, sprinkle seaweed, bonito flakes and enjoy the taste.

Nutritional Information

- Preparation Time: 30 minutes
- Total servings: 2
- Calories: 489(per serving)
- Fat: 46.2g
- Protein: 4.17g
- Carbs: 11.23g

Cheesy Hamm

Ingredients

- Ham 4 oz.
- Mozzarella cheese 5 oz.
- Cheddar cheese 3.5 oz.
- Mascarpone cheese 3 oz.
- Coconut flour 4 tbsp.
- Almond Flour 3 tbsp.
- Egg 1
- Italian seasoning 1 tsp.
- Salt and pepper to taste

Preparation Method

- At first, preheat the oven to 400F and in a microwave or toaster oven, melt your mozzarella cheese. About 1 minute in the microwave, and 10-second intervals afterward, or about 10 minutes in an oven, stirring occasionally.
- In a mixing bowl, mix almond, coconut flour, seasonings, salt, pepper, mozzarella (melted), mascarpone, egg and make moist dough, transfer it to a flat surface with some parchment paper.
- Using rolling pin flatten dough and using knife cut diagonal lines beginning from the edges of the dough to the center, leave a row of dough untouched about 4 inches wide.

- Alternate lay ham and cheddar on that uncut stretch of dough then cover your filling by lift one section of dough at a time and lay it over the top.
- Finally, bake in preheated oven for 20 minutes until you see it has turned a golden brown color and enjoy the taste.

Nutritional Information

- Preparation Time: 40 minutes
- Total servings: 4
- Calories: 306 (per serving)
- Fat: 35.7g
- Protein: 24.5g
- Carbs: 4.7g

Spinach Quiche

Ingredients

- Ghee 1 tbsp.
- Onion 1 oz.
- Frozen chopped spinach 10 oz.
- Eggs 8
- 3 cups shredded raw cheese 10 oz.
- Mascarpone cheese 2 oz.
- Sea salt 1 tsp.
- Black pepper 1/2 tsp.

Preparation Method

- At first, preheat your oven to 350F and place your pan over medium heat. When ghee is hot, add onions and cook until it becomes soft.
- Add spinach and cook for 2 minutes and keep aside. In a bowl, mix egg, cheese, mascarpone, salt, pepper and add to spinach mixture.
- Using blender, blend the mixture and pour into pan, place in preheated oven for 30 minutes and enjoy the taste.

Nutritional Information

- Preparation Time: 40 minutes
- Total servings: 4
- Calories: 588.25 (per serving)

- Fat: 48.2g
- Protein: 32.4g
- Carbs: 5.2g

Chicken Pizza

Ingredients

- Chicken breast 0.3 lb. (skinless and boneless)
- Ghee 1 tbsp.
- Garlic clove 1
- Heavy whipping cream 4 oz.
- Mascarpone cheese 2 oz.
- Fresh spinach 4 oz.
- Shredded mozzarella 2 oz.
- Sea salt and pepper to taste
- Fathead pizza dough 1

Preparation Method

- At first, wash and cut the chicken breast piece into small pieces.
- Place a pan over medium heat with ghee, when ghee is hot, add chicken breast pieces and cook for 10 minutes, keep aside.
- Add garlic, cream to pan, when sauce starts to thicken, add spinach and cook just until wilted.
- Spread sauce and spinach mixture onto to pizza crust; add shredded cheese, mascarpone, and chicken.
- Place in oven and bake for 5 minutes at 350F or until cheese is melted completely.

Nutritional Information

- Preparation Time: 8 minutes
- Total servings: 2
- Calories: 473.5 (per serving)
- Fat: 40.1g
- Protein: 22.1g
- Carbs: 6.1g

Coconut Meatball

Ingredients
Meatballs

- Ghee 1 tbsp.
- Ground beef 0.5lb
- Onions 1 oz.
- Garlic cloves 2
- Coconut flour 1.2 oz.
- Coconut milk 1 tbsp.
- Salt to taste

Coconut Broth

- Coconut milk 2 oz.
- Broth 2 oz.

Spices

- Coriander seeds 1 tsp.
- Turmeric 1/2 tsp.
- Cinnamon 1/2 tsp.
- Red pepper 1/2 tsp.
- Lemongrass 1/2 tsp.
- Fresh ginger 1/2 tsp.
- Lime zest 1/2 tsp.

Preparation Method

- In a large pan, add ghee. When ghee is hot, add garlic, onions and cook until fragrant and translucent.
- Meantime, combine coconut flour, coconut milk, ground beef, salt and create a paste.
- Add onions, garlic to this paste and create small balls using hand.
- Place the pan over medium heat and add ghee. When ghee is hot add meatballs all over the pan (approximately 15 minutes).
- When meat are browned on both sides, add coconut milk, broth, and all spices, mix well and cook for 20 more minutes.
- Finally, serve with some coconut broth with meatballs in a bowl and enjoy the taste.

Nutritional Information

- Preparation Time: 30 minutes
- Total servings: 2
- Calories: 566 (per serving)
- Fat: 47.5g
- Protein: 24g
- Carbs: 4g

Sausage Bacon

Ingredients
- Sausages 6
- Bacon 12 slices
- Cheddar Cheese 1 oz.
- Mascarpone cheese 1 oz.
- Swiss Cheese 2 oz.
- Garlic Powder ½ tsp.
- Onion Powder ½ tsp.
- Salt and Pepper to taste

Preparation Method
- Preheat oven to 400F. Make a slit in all of the sausage to make room for the cheese.
- Slice swiss cheese, mascarpone and cheddar cheese from a block into small long rectangles and stuff into the sausage.
- Start by tightly wrapping one slice of bacon around the sausage. Continue tightly wrapping the second slice of bacon around the sausage, slightly overlapping with the first slice.
- Poke toothpicks through each side of the bacon and sausage, securing the bacon in place. Set on a wire rack that's on top of a cookie sheet. Season with garlic powder, onion powder, salt and pepper.

- Bake for 40 minutes, or until bacon is crispy. Additionally broil the bacon on top if needed. Serve up with some delicious creamed spinach.

Nutritional Information

- Preparation Time: 45 minutes
- Serving per Recipe: 6
- Calories:437.6 (per serving)
- Fat: 39.9g
- Protein: 19.6g
- Carbs: 2.6g

Chicken Zoodles Box

Ingredients
- Chicken legs 3.5 oz.
- Butter 1 tbsp.
- Ghee 1tbsp.
- Curry powder ½ tsp.
- Spring onion 1 stalk
- Garlic 1 clove
- Large egg 1
- Sprouts 1 oz.
- Zucchini 3.5 oz.
- Soy sauce 1 tsp.
- Fish sauce ½ tsp.
- Pepper ¼ tsp.
- Lime juice 1 tsp.
- Green chilies 1
- Cilantro 1 tbsp.
- Salt and pepper to taste

Preparation Method
- Season the chicken with curry powder, salt and pepper and keep aside.
- Prepare the sauce by combining soy sauce, fish sauce. Finely chop spring onion, garlic and make zoodles out of zucchini (use spiralizer).

- Fry the seasoned chicken with butter until brown. In a pan, melt ghee and chopped spring onion until fragrant and add garlic, egg into the pan.
- Add sprouts and zoodles and mix everything well together. Add sauce and stir and reduce until there is little liquid left.
- Add fried chicken pieces and stir and garnish with a few chopped green chilies, cilantro and squeeze some lemon juice on top. Serve and enjoy the taste.

Nutritional Information

- Preparation Time: 20 minutes
- Total servings: 1
- Calories: 606 (per serving)
- Fat: 48.2g
- Protein: 24.2g
- Carbs: 6.9g

Tomato Frittata

Ingredients

- Large eggs 6
- Red onion 2 oz.
- Feta cheese 3.5 oz.
- Mascarpone cheese 2 oz.
- Cherry tomatoes 3.5 oz.
- Ghee 1 tbsp.
- Herbs 2 tbsp.
- Salt and pepper to taste

Preparation Method

- At first, preheat the oven 400F. Place a large skillet over medium heat and add ghee, when ghee is hot add chopped red onions .
- Now, whisk eggs into a separate bowl with salt and pepper. Add finely chopped herbs and whisk well until it combines.
- When the onion is lightly browned, pour the egg mixture into skillet and cook until you see the edges turning dark.
- Top with the crumbled cheese (feta and mascarpone) and halved cherry tomatoes and place in preheated oven for 5 minutes or until the top is cooked.
- Remove from the oven and set aside to cool down for 2 minutes. Serve and enjoy the taste.

Nutritional Information

- Preparation Time: 15 minutes
- Total servings: 2
- Calories: 435 (per serving)
- Fat: 40g
- Protein: 26g
- Carbs: 6g

Keto Lunch

Ingredients

- Large eggs 2
- Parmesan cheese 1 oz.
- Fresh basil 1 tbsp.
- Fresh oregano ½ tbsp..
- Ghee 2 tbsp.
- Salt and pepper to taste
- Avocado 1.8 oz.
- Bacon 1 oz. (crisped)

Preparation Method

- At first, grate the Parmesan cheese and keep aside.
- Next, crack the eggs into a small bowl and add chopped herbs and Parmesan cheese.
- Keep large skillet over medium heat and add ghee, when ghee is hot, pour the egg mixture in and decrease the heat and cook for 1 minute each side.
- When omelet is ready, place on a serving plate and top with crisped up bacon and sliced avocado pieces.

Nutritional Information

- Preparation Time: 10 minutes
- Total servings: 2

- Calories: 359.5 (per serving)
- Fat: 31.65g
- Protein: 8.55g
- Carbs: 1.65g

Zucchini Bacon Fry

Ingredients

- Zucchini 7 oz.
- Bacon 2 oz.
- Red onion 1 oz.
- Garlic clove 1
- Ghee 1 tbsp.
- Fresh parsley 1 tbsp.
- Salt ¼ tsp.

Preparation Method

- At first, chop red onion, garlic, bacon and add it to large skillet over a medium heat and cook until it turns light brown color.
- On the other hand, dice the zucchini into medium cube size pieces and add to skillet, cook for 15 minutes. Don't forget to stir frequently and finally add chopped parsley.

Nutritional Information

- Preparation Time: 25 minutes
- Total servings: 1
- Calories: 422 (per serving)
- Fat: 35.5g
- Protein: 17.4g
- Carbs: 6.6g

Salmon Wraps

Ingredients

- Large eggs 3
- Avocado 3.5 oz.
- Smoked salmon 1.8 oz.
- Cream cheese 2 tbsp.
- Fresh chives 2 tbsp.
- Spring onion 2 tbsp.
- Ghee 1 tbsp.
- Salt and pepper to taste

Preparation Method

- At first, whisk egg, salt, pepper in a small bowl, add cream cheese with chopped chives and keep aside.
- Place pan over medium heat and add ghee. When ghee is hot, add egg mixture into pan and cook for 1 minute each side .Meanwhile, slice the smoked salmon, avocado and keep aside.
- Now, place the omelet on a plate and add sliced salmon, avocado and fold into a wrap.

Nutritional Information

- Preparation Time: 15 minutes
- Total servings: 2
- Calories: 382.5 (per serving)

- Fat: 33.45g
- Protein: 18.5g
- Carbs: 2.9g

Slim Lunch

Ingredients

- Egg 1
- Bacon slices 2 (2.3 oz.)
- Mushrooms 6 oz.
- Avocado 3.5 oz.
- Ghee 1 tbsp.
- Salt and pepper to taste
- Fresh herbs (garnish)

Preparation Method

- In a small pan, roast the mushrooms with ghee and season with salt, pepper. Keep aside.
- Now, roast the bacon and keep aside. In the same pan, make an omelet with egg and garnish with freshly chopped herbs.
- Meanwhile, slice the avocado and place all items on serving plate and enjoy the taste.

Nutritional Information

- Preparation Time: 15 minutes
- Total servings: 1
- Calories: 489 (per serving)
- Fat: 41g
- Protein: 20g
- Carbs: 6.6g

Rind Quiche

Ingredients

Crust

- Pork rinds 5.3 oz.
- Coconut flour 5.3 oz.
- Flax meal 3 tbsp. (60 g / 2.1 oz)
- Large eggs 3
- Himalayan salt 1/2 tsp.

Filling

- Large eggs 6
- Heavy whipping cream 4 fl oz.
- Spring onions 1 oz.
- Shredded cheddar cheese 7 oz.
- Shredded mascarpone cheese 4 oz.
- Cream cheese 8.8 oz.
- Asparagus spears 8.8 oz.
- Salt and pepper to taste
- Fresh herbs for garnish
- Ghee 1 tbsp.

Preparation Method

- At first, preheat the oven to 400F. Put the pork rinds into a food processor or blender and make powder out of pork rinds.

- Add powdered rind in a mixing bowl together with the coconut flour and flax meal, Himalaya salt and mix until well combined.
- Now, crack the eggs and mix the dough using hand or hand mixer, place this dough in a rectangular baking tray with removable bottom (30 x 20 cm / 12 x 8 inch).
- Bake in preheated oven for 15 minutes and keep aside until it cools down. Reduce the oven to 350F.
- Now, add shredded cheese's (cheddar and mascarpone) over cooled crust and keep aside.
- Meantime, take a large bowl and crack the eggs, add the cream, season with salt and pepper and whisk until it combines well.
- On the other hand, place a pan over medium heat with ghee. When ghee is hot, add sliced spring onions and cook for 3 minutes or until fragrant. Add this to the egg mixture and combine well.
- Add cream cheese to egg mixture and pour over shredded cheese. Now, top egg mixture with asparagus and place in preheated oven for 30 minutes or until lightly browned and crispy on top.
- Garnish with freshly chopped herbs and enjoy the taste.

Nutritional Information

- Preparation Time: 60 minutes
- Total servings: 8
- Calories: 660 (per serving)
- Fat: 51.45g
- Protein: 39g
- Carbs: 4.2g

Dinner Recipes

Green Salmon

Ingredients

- Salmon fillets 1 lb.
- Fresh chopped lavender leaves 2 tbsp.
- Macadamia nuts 1 oz.
- Maple syrup 1 tbsp.
- Mustard ½ tsp.
- Dill ¼ tsp.
- Butter 1 tbsp.
- Salt and pepper to taste

Preparation Method

- Preheat the oven to 350F. Add macadamia nuts, lavender, maple syrup, your spices and mustard in food processor and make a paste.
- Heat the pan and add ghee and fry dry salmon fillets for about 3 minutes.
- Add the paste to the top side of salmon fillets. Once they seared, transfer them to an oven and bake for about 10 minutes.
- Serve with some fresh baby spinach and little smoked paprika. Enjoy the taste.

Nutritional Information

- Preparation Time: 15 minutes

- Serving per Recipe: 2
- Calories: 397 (per serving)
- Fat: 44.2g
- Protein: 19.1g
- Carbohydrates: 5g

Cheesy Sandwich Cream

Ingredients

- Zucchini 35 oz.
- Mozzarella 8 oz.
- Mascarpone cheese 2 oz.
- Ghee 1 tbsp.
- Garlic 1 clove
- Salt and black pepper to taste
- Cooked prawns 1 oz.
- Almond butter 1 tbsp.
- Fresh basil 2 tbsp.
- Cream ½ cup

Preparation Method

- At first, preheat oven at 450F. Slice a thin slice each zucchini into 3 pieces and place in a flat frying pan or a baked sheet.
- Apply ghee to zcchini. Season with salt, pepper and sprinkle chopped garlic over the zucchini. Fry until softened and heated by, about 15 minutes.
- Meanwhile, cut the mozzarella, mascarpone, prawns into six ½-inch thick slices. Using a spatula, sandwich each slice between 2 hot zucchini halves and apply almond butter and cream.
- Before serving, garnish with basil and enjoy the taste.

Nutritional Information

- Preparation Time: 20 minutes
- Total servings: 6 pieces
- Calories: 255.7 (per serving)
- Fat: 19.8g
- Protein: 9.9g
- Carbs: 4.88g

Vegetable Stew

Ingredients

- Vegetable mix 1 lb.
- Ghee 2 tbsp.
- Onion powder 1 ½ tbsp..
- Garlic powder 1 ½ tsp.
- Ginger powder 1 tsp.
- Tomato puree 1.5 oz.
- All spice 1 ½ tbsp..
- Smoked paprika 1 ½ tsp.
- Salt to taste
- Diced tomatoes 7 oz.
- Heavy cream ½ cup
- Coconut milk 1 cup
- Almond butter 1 tbsp.
- Cashew butter 1 tbsp.
- Cilantro 1 ½ tbsp.
- Topping: Sharp grated cheese 1 tbsp. for each serving

Preparation Method

- At first, mix chopped vegetables into bite sized pieces and season with salt, pepper and ground pepper, ginger and mix well.

- Add canned diced tomatoes and tomato paste, mix well again. Finally, add coconut milk, cashew butter and mix well.
- Starts cooking for 35 minutes on medium heat, after 25 minutes, add heavy cream and mix thoroughly.
- Before serving, add ghee, cheese and enjoy the taste.

Nutritional Information

- Preparation Time: 40 minutes
- Serving per Recipe: 5
- Calories: 543.6 (per serving)
- Fat: 40.7g
- Protein: 22.7g
- Carbs: 6g

Cheese Filled Onions

Ingredients

- Onions 8 oz.
- Ghee 1 ½ tbsp..
- Mascarpone cheese 2 oz.
- Mozzarella cheese 1 oz. (small balls)
- Coconut cream 2 oz.
- Beef meat 1 oz.
- Prawns 1 oz.
- Salt and black pepper to taste

Preparation Method

- At first, in large e skillet, add half ghee. When ghee is hot, add chopped beef, prawns and cook for 10 minutes.
- On the other hand, remove middle flesh of onions and lace in baking tray with the remaining ghee and salt and pepper.
- Add cooked meat. Layer cheese and coconut cream as topping and shake the onion occasionally, cook until it is tender and slightly charred in oven for minimum 15 minutes.

Nutritional Information

- Preparation Time: 30 minutes
- Total servings: 4

- Calories: 186.2 (per serving)
- Fat: 14.8g
- Protein: 6.1g
- Carbs: 3g

Walnut Tuna

Ingredients
- Walnuts 30g
- Raw honey 15g
- Mustard 3g
- Dill 2g
- Tuna fillets 550g
- Olive oil 14g
- Salt and pepper to taste

Preparation Method
- Preheat the oven to 350F. Add walnuts, raw honey, your spices and mustard in the kitchen machine and make a paste.
- Heat the pan and add olive oil and fry dry tuna fillets for about 3 minutes. Add the walnut paste to the top of the tuna fillets.
- Once fried, transfer them to an oven and bake for about 10 minutes. Serve with a little fresh baby kale and a little smoked paprika. Enjoy the delicious taste.

Nutritional Information
- Preparation Time: 15 minutes
- Total servings: 2

- Calories: 373 (per serving)
- Fat: 43g
- Protein: 20g
- Carbs: 3g

Chicken Squash Noodles

Ingredients

- Summer squash 100g
- Curry Powder 4g
- Chicken legs 100g
- Purified butter 15g
- Coconut oil 14g
- Spring onion 1 stem
- Garlic 1 clove
- Egg 1
- Beans sprout 35g
- Coconut milk 50g
- Soy sauce 5g
- Oyster sauce 2g
- White pepper 3g
- Lemon juice 5g
- Red Chili peppers 1
- Salt and pepper to taste

Preparation Method

- Season the chicken with curry powder, salt and pepper and set aside. Prepare the sauce by combining soy sauce, oyster sauce.

- Cut the onion, mince the garlic and remove the ingredients from the squash (use the spiralizer). Fry the spiced chicken with butter until brown.
- In a pan, melt coconut oil and chopped spring onion until fragrant and add garlic, egg into the pan. Add bean sprouts and zoodles and mix well.
- Add coconut milk, sauce and stir and reduce until little liquid is left. Add fried chicken pieces and stir and garnish with a few chopped red chilies and squeeze some lemon juice on top. Serve while hot.

Nutritional Information

- Preparation Time: 20 minutes
- Total servings: 1
- Calories: 673 (per serving)
- Fat: 57.8g
- Protein: 27.1g
- Carbs: 7.9g

Roasted Asparagus Meat

Ingredients

- Asparagus 225g (trimmed)
- Ghee 20g
- Mascarpone cheese 56g
- Feta cheese 28g (cubes)
- Coconut cream 50g
- Pork rib meat 28g
- Minced shrimp 28g
- Salt and black pepper to taste

Preparation Method

- At first, in large e skillet, add ghee 10g. When ghee is hot, add chopped pork, shrimp and cook for 10 minutes.
- On the other hand, in baking tray, dice the asparagus with the remaining ghee and salt and pepper.
- Brush the asparagus in a single layer and add cooked meat. Layer cheese and coconut cream as topping and shake the baking tray occasionally, until it is tender and slightly charred, 15 minutes.

Nutritional Information

- Preparation Time: 30 minutes
- Total servings: 4

- Calories: 186.25 (per serving)
- Fat: 16.10g
- Protein: 6.32g
- Carbs: 3.3g

Tofu Chicken

Ingredients
- Chicken leg 1300g
- Tofu 200g
- Water 240 ml
- Crushed tomatoes 40g
- Heavy whipped cream 40g
- Ghee 35g
- Olive oil 10g
- Coconut oil 20g
- Garlic paste 6g
- Ginger paste 6g
- Coriander powder 4g
- Allspice 4g
- Salt and pepper to taste
- Red chili powder 4g
- Coriander 5 springs

Preparation Method
- Preheat the oven to 375F, add olive oil to the chicken, taste the salt, pepper and place the marinated chicken in the oven for 25 minutes.
- Cut tofu into small cubes pieces and set aside and heat the pan over medium heat and add ghee, coconut oil. When the

ghee starts to brown, add ginger, garlic and mix for 2 minutes.

- Add tomato, coriander powder, allspice, red chili powder and salt. Mix well all together, adding tofu into boiling sauce.
- Add water and let it simmer for 5 minutes and add cream, slowly stir in the medium heat. Add chicken pieces gently into the sauce and let it boil for 5 minutes.
- Garnish with coriander and enjoy the taste.

Nutritional Information

- Preparation Time: 35 minutes
- Total servings: 4
- Calories: 490 (per serving)
- Fat: 44.1g
- Protein: 17.4g
- Carbs: 4.2g

Asparagus Frittata

Ingredients

- Large eggs 10
- Asparagus spears 8.8 oz. (20 pieces)
- Spring onions 0.4 oz.
- Shallot 0.7 oz.
- Red bell pepper 5.3 oz.
- Heavy whipping cream 2 fl oz.
- Fresh goat cheese 5.3 oz.
- Pancetta 3.5 oz. (alternative bacon)
- Fresh parsley 2 tbsp.
- Fresh mint 2 tbsp.
- Fresh tarragon 1 tbsp.
- Ghee 2 tbsp.
- Salt and pepper to taste

Preparation Method

- At first, preheat your oven to 400F. Before we start cooking, slice asparagus by cutting the ends, bell pepper into small stripes, shallot, spring onion and keep aside.
- Place pan over medium heat and add ghee. When ghee is hot add all diced ingredients into pan, salt and cook for 5 minutes and keep aside in baking dish.
- In a small bowl, whisk the eggs, cream, chopped parsley, mint, salt, black pepper and keep aside.

- Crumble the soft goat cheese all over the vegetables and pour the egg mixture over it and place in preheated oven for 20 minutes just until the top becomes firm.
- After that lay the pancetta (or bacon) all over it and place back in the oven for another 15 minutes. Serve warm and enjoy the taste.

Nutritional Information

- Preparation Time: 60 minutes
- Total servings: 4
- Calories: 503 (per serving)
- Fat: 38g
- Protein: 25.5g
- Carbs: 6g

Casserole Dinner

Ingredients

- Sausage meat 1.1 lb.
- Red onion 3.9 oz.
- Garlic cloves 3
- Diced pumpkin 8.2 oz.
- Dijon mustard 1 tbsp.
- Shredded cheddar cheese 8 oz.
- Large eggs 6
- Heavy whipping cream 4 fl oz.
- Ghee 3 tbsp.
- Salt and pepper to taste
- Sriracha sauce for topping

Preparation Method

- At first, preheat your oven to 350F. Place large pan over medium heat and add ghee. When ghee is hot, add sausage meat and break all large pieces.
- Cook until the meat is browned from all sides, about 10 minutes and add to the large mixing bowl and keep aside.
- Now, slice red onion, garlic and cook in the same pan which is used to cook sausage until fragrant and lightly browned, about 10 minutes.
- Dice the pumpkin into cube pieces, add to the pan and cook for 10 minutes. When it cools down, add to the meat bowl

and add mustard, shredded cheddar cheese and mix until well combined (save little cheese for topping purpose).
- Crack the eggs in a small bowl and mix with the cream, salt, pepper and pour in mixing bowl. Top with the remaining cheddar cheese and place in preheated oven for 25 minutes or until the top is golden brown. Just before serving, add Sriracha sauce on top and enjoy the taste.

Nutritional Information

- Preparation Time: 50 minutes
- Total servings: 6
- Calories: 577 (per serving)
- Fat: 47.3g
- Protein: 30.5g
- Carbs: 6g

Tuna Colcannon

Ingredients

- Ghee 2 tbsp.
- Bacon 8.5 oz.
- Shredded tuna 3 oz.
- Cauliflower 1.3 lb.
- Green cabbage 10.6 oz.
- Spring onions 2 oz.
- Heavy whipping cream 4 fl oz.
- Salt and pepper to taste
- Freshly chopped parsley for garnish

Preparation Method

- At first, place a large saucepan over medium heat and add ghee. When ghee is hot, add bacon slices and tuna and cook for 10 minutes or until crisped up and keep aside.
- Meanwhile, slice the cabbage, cauliflower, spring onions and add to pan, cook for another 10 minutes or until it looks tender.
- Finally, season with salt, pepper, cream and freshly chopped herbs. If desire, before serving add little ghee and enjoy the taste.

Nutritional Information

- Preparation Time: 30 minutes

- Total servings: 6
- Calories: 363 (per serving)
- Fat: 30.7g
- Protein:13 g
- Carbs: 5.5g

Wild Cheesy Sausage

Ingredients

- Sausage 1.5 oz.
- Onion 1 tablespoon
- Wild mushrooms 2 oz.
- Parmesan cheese 0.5 oz.
- Mascarpone cheese 1 oz.
- Mozzarella 0.5 oz.
- Oregano 1 tsp.
- Basil 1 tsp.
- Salt 1/2 tsp.
- Red pepper 1/2 tsp.
- Ghee 1 tbsp.

Preparation Method

- At first, preheat the oven to 350F. Place the skillet over medium heat and ghee.
- When ghee is hot, add sausage, cook for 15 minutes and keep aside.
- Meanwhile, slice wild mushrooms (or forest mushrooms), onion and cook in skillet until it turns to golden brown color.
- Now, cut sausages into round slices and put back in skillet, add parmesan cheese, mascarpone cheese and stir once.

- Your skillet into preheated oven for 15 minutes before you remove sprinkle grated mozzarella cheese and herbs. Let it cool for 10 minutes and enjoy the taste.

Nutritional Information

- Preparation Time: 25 minutes
- Total servings: 1
- Calories: 630 (per serving)
- Fat: 51 g
- Protein: 30g
- Carbs: 5g

Crepes with Blueberries

Ingredients

- Cream cheese 2 oz.
- Large eggs 2
- Stevia 10 drops
- Cinnamon 1/4 tsp.
- Baking soda 1/4 tsp.
- Salt 1/8 tsp.
- Ghee 1 tbsp.

Filling

- Cream cheese 4 oz.
- Vanillas extract 1/2 tsp.
- Erythritol 2 tbsp.
- Blueberries 2 oz.

Preparation Method

- In a small bowl, add cream cheese, eggs and mix using hand mixer until it becomes completely smooth.
- Add stevia, cinnamon, baking soda, salt and combine well. Place a nonstick pan over a medium heat and ghee. When ghee is hot add butter (1/4 cup at a time) and cook for 2 minutes both sides or until edges become crispy.

- Meanwhile, prepare to fill by combining all filling ingredients in a bowl and mix using hand mixer until it becomes creamy paste.
- When the crepes is cooked, spread filling over crepes and top with blueberries and fold it and enjoy with little cream over it.

Nutritional Information

- Preparation Time: 35 minutes
- Total servings: 2
- Calories: 390 (per serving)
- Fat: 32g
- Protein: 14.1g
- Carbs: 7g

Spicy Tuna Bowl

Ingredients

- Fresh tuna 0.5 lb.
- Soy sauce 1 tbsp.
- Sesame oil 2 tsp.
- Avocados 1 oz.
- Edamame 2 oz.
- Macadamia nuts 1 oz. (crushed)
- Mozzarella 1 oz. (grated)
- Noodle rice 2 oz.
- Scallion 1 oz.
- Jalapeno 2 tbsp.
- Sarayo sauce 2 tbsp.
- Salt and pepper to taste
- Mayonnaise 2 tbsp.
- Sriracha sauce 1 tbsp.
- Lime juice 1 tbsp.
- Black and white sesame seeds 1 tbsp. (roasted)

Preparation Method

- At first, Add cooked tuna chunks to small bowl and add soy sauce, sesame oil, marinate and keep in fridge for at least 60 minutes.
- Meanwhile, make noodle rice by boiling for 2 minutes in hot water and remove water, keep aside.

- In a mixing bowl, add avocado chunks, shelled edamame, noodle rice, chopped scallion, jalapeno, macadamia nuts and mix well.
- Now, add marinated tuna, sarayo sauce and mix well. Finally, top with mayonnaise, sriracha, lime juice, salt, pepper and gently combine.
- Before serving garnish with mozzarella, roasted sesame seeds and enjoy the taste.

Nutritional Information

- Preparation Time: 75 minutes
- Total servings: 2
- Calories: 483.2 (per serving)
- Fat: 43g
- Protein: 28g
- Carbs: 8g

Soup Recipes

Chicken Bone Soup

Ingredients

- Chicken bone 1.2 lb.
- Onion Powder 1 tsp.
- Garlic Powder 1 tsp.
- Celery Seed ½ tsp.
- Ginger powder 1 tsp.
- Chili powder ½ tsp.
- Ghee 2 oz.
- Squash 1 oz.
- Soy sauce 2 oz.
- Chicken broth 3 cups
- Cream 1 cup
- Cream cheese 2 oz.
- Salt and Pepper to taste

Preparation Method

- Cut or slice the chicken bones into chunks and drop them in the pot and add all the rest of the ingredients to the cooking pot except cream, cheese.
- Set cooking pots on heat for 60 minutes and cook completely. Once everything is cooked, remove the chicken from the cooking pot and shred using a fork.
- Add cream and cheese to the cooking pot. Using an immersion blender, emulsify all of the liquids together.

This will help the soup from separating while you are eating.

- Place the chicken back into the cooking pot and add cooked squash, stir together. Taste and season with extra salt, pepper, and soy sauce. Serve and enjoy the taste.

Nutritional Information

- Preparation Time: 190 minutes
- Serving per Recipe: 5
- Calories:541.2 (per serving)
- Fat: 45g
- Protein: 21g
- Carbs: 4.5g

Bacon Soup

Ingredients

- Vegetable broth 1 ½ cups
- Bacon 4 slices
- Pumpkin puree 1 cup
- Ghee 1 oz.
- Butter 1 oz.
- White onion 2 oz.
- Garlic cloves 2
- Salt ½ tsp.
- Pepper ½ tsp.
- Red chili flakes 2
- Fresh ginger ½ tsp.
- Coriander ¼ tsp.
- Bay Leaf 1
- Cream ½ cup

Preparation Method

- Keep saucepan over medium heat, add ghee. When ghee is hot, add garlic and fresh ginger.
- Once the ghee has turned a dark golden color, add onion, garlic, and ginger to the pan and stir well. Let this sauté for about 3 minutes or until onions start to go translucent.
- Once onions are translucent, add spices (salt, pepper, coriander, bay leaf, red chili flakes) to the pan and let cook

for 2 minutes. Add pumpkin puree to pan and stir into the onions and spices well.

- Once the pumpkin is mixed well, add vegetable broth to the pan. Stir until everything is combined.
- Bring to a boil to simmer for 20 minutes. Once simmered, use an immersion blender to blend together all of the ingredients. You want a smooth puree here so make sure you take your time. Cook for an additional 20 minutes.
- In the meantime, cook 4 slices of bacon over medium heat. Once the soup is ready, pour in cream and the grease from the cooked bacon and mix well.
- Crumble the bacon over the top of the soup and enjoy the taste of the soup.

Nutritional Information

- Preparation Time: 45 minutes
- Serving per Recipe: 3
- Calories:489.7 (per serving)
- Fat: 44.6g
- Protein: 10.9g
- Carbs: 4.9g

Green Beef Soup

Ingredients
- Ground beef 1lb.
- Sausage 7.1 oz.
- Green beans 7.1 oz.
- Tomatoes 14.1 oz. (tin)
- Fresh tomatoes 7.1 oz.
- Tomato Puree 2.2 oz.
- Red chilies 1.1 oz.
- Red pepper 4.2 oz.
- White onion 3.9 oz.
- Garlic cloves 2
- Tabasco sauce 1 tbsp.
- Ghee 4 tbsp.
- Salt and pepper to taste
- Water 1 liter
- Fresh cilantro and parsley for garnish

Preparation Method
- At first, dice the onion, garlic. Halve, red pepper, red chili peppers, sausage, tomatoes, green beans and keep aside.
- Place large Dutch pan over medium heat with ghee. Once ghee hot, add the diced onion, garlic and cook 2 minutes or until lightly browned, then add the sliced red pepper, red

chili peppers and cook for 5 minutes, don't forget to stir to prevent burning.

- Add the sausage, ground beef into the pot and cook until it turns to brown color. Add the chopped tomatoes, tinned tomatoes, tomato puree and tabasco sauce to taste.
- Now, add water, beans and season with salt and pepper. Cook the soup until bubbles appears and before serving, add chopped cilantro and parsley.

Nutritional Information

- Preparation Time: 30 minutes
- Total servings: 8
- Calories: 371 (per serving)
- Fat: 29.5g
- Protein: 18.5g
- Carbs: 6.5g

Cheesy Pork Soup

Ingredients

- Pork Sausage 2 lb.
- Pork stock 4 cups
- Ghee 2 tsp.
- Kale 5 oz.
- Onion Powder 1 tsp.
- Chili powder 1 tsp.
- Cumin 1 tsp.
- Garlic Powder 1 tsp.
- Salt ½ tsp.
- Basil 2 tbsp.
- Cheese 3 oz.

Preparation Method

- Heat ghee in a large pot over medium heat. Once hot, add sausage to the pan, allow it to cook slightly.
- As the sausage cooks, add sliced green pepper into pieces, season with salt and pepper.
- Add the tomatoes and stir. Then, add the spinach on top of everything and place the lid on the pot.
- Cook until spinach is wilted, about 6 minutes. In the meantime, measure out all spices and grab your beef stock to have handy.

- Once the spinach is wilted, mix it together with the sausage. Then add the spices and mix again. Lastly, add the broth and mix once again.
- Reduce the heat to medium and cook for 30 minutes. Reduce the heat to simmer and cook 15 more minutes. Before serving, add basil and enjoy the flavor.

Nutritional Information

- Preparation Time: 55 minutes
- Serving per Recipe: 6
- Calories:501.6 (per serving)
- Fat: 40.6g
- Protein: 23.2g
- Carbs: 4.6g

Hot Creamy Soup

Ingredients

- Vegetable broth 1 ½ cup
- 2 Chicken Bouillon
- Cream 2 tbsp.
- Ghee 1 tbsp.
- Eggs 2
- Parsley 2 tbsp.
- Chili ½ tsp.
- Garlic Paste ½ tsp.

Preparation Method

- Place a pan over medium heat and add vegetable broth, bouillon cube, and ghee.
- Bring the broth to a boil and stir everything together. Then, add the chili, garlic paste and stir again. Turn the stove off.
- Beat the eggs in a separate container and pour into the steaming broth, cream. Stir together well and let sit for a moment and add chopped parsley leaves. Serve up some awesome tasting soup in 5 minutes.

Nutritional Information

- Preparation Time: 5 minutes
- Serving per Recipe: 1

- Calories:300 (per serving)
- Fat: 27.7g
- Protein: 12.9g
- Carbs: 4.4g

Chicken Cheese Soup

Ingredients

- Chicken 4.4 lb.
- White onion 3.5 oz.
- Garlic cloves 4
- Tomatoes 14.1 oz.
- Green beans 14.1 oz.
- BBQ Sauce 6 oz.
- Shredded mozzarella cheese 6 oz.
- Shredded mascarpone cheese 4 oz.
- Ghee 2 oz.
- Chicken stock 2 liters
- Salt and pepper to taste
- Fresh herbs for garnish

Preparation Method

- At first, Boil the chicken for 60 minutes in water, after cooking shredded chicken and keep aside.
- Place large pan over medium heat with ghee. When ghee is hot, add sliced onion, garlic and cook until lightly browned and fragrant. Add chicken stock and bring to a boil over a high heat for 15 minutes.
- Meanwhile, cut green beans and add to the pot including tomatoes. Cook another 15 minutes.

- Now, add BBQ sauce and shredded chicken and turn off the heat. Season with salt and pepper.
- Grate the mozzarella cheese, mascarpone cheese and chopped herbs over soup and serve warm to enjoy the delicious taste.

Nutritional Information

- Preparation Time: 90 minutes
- Total servings: 8
- Calories: 514 (per serving)
- Fat: 40.5g
- Protein: 30g
- Carbs: 7g

Gnocchi Sausage Soup

Ingredients

- Ground Italian sausage 1 lb.
- Keto garlic gnocchi 3 oz.
- Red onion 2.5 oz.
- Garlic cloves 2
- Beef bone broth 1 liter
- Red pepper 4.2 oz.
- Chopped kale 2.4 oz.
- Heavy cream 4 fl oz.
- Salt and black pepper to taste
- Ghee 2 tbsp

Preparation Method

- Place Dutch oven over medium heat and add ghee. When ghee is hot, add sausage, onion, garlic and cook until the sausage is completely browned, don't forget to stir occasionally to avoid burns.
- Add in the beef bone broth, red peppers to the pot and decrease the heat to low.
- Now, add the kale and cook another 5 minutes. Add gnocchi, cream and stir until it combines well.
- Now, season with salt and pepper. If desired, garnish with chopped fresh herbs.

Nutritional Information

- Preparation Time: 30 minutes
- Total servings: 4
- Calories: 691(per serving)
- Fat: 56g
- Protein: 38g
- Carbs: 88g

Pepper Chicken Soup

Ingredients
- Ghee 2 tbsp.
- Red onion 4 oz.
- Shredded chicken breast 17.6 oz.
- Chicken broth 1.5l
- Water 500 ml
- Heavy cream 4 fl oz.
- Mascarpone cheese 4 oz.
- Macadamia nuts powder 1 oz.
- Lemon juice 3 tbsp.
- Cauliflower 15 oz. (riced)
- Large eggs 3
- Salt and pepper to taste
- Herbs for garnish

Preparation Method
- At first, rice the cauliflower using food processor and keep aside.
- Place a large pan over medium heat with ghee. When ghee is hot, add onions and cook until translucent and turning light brown color.
- Add your chicken broth, water, cream, shredded chicken, rice cauliflower, herbs, lemon juice and cook for 10 minutes to allow the cauliflower to become tender.

- Meanwhile, beat 3 eggs together in a small bowl and slowly add to the soup and decrease the heat to low and cook for 10 minutes.
- Now, add shredded mascarpone cheese and macadamia powder and stir for a few minutes. Turn off heat and serve immediately with some freshly chopped herbs.

Nutritional Information

- Preparation Time: 30 minutes
- Total servings: 8
- Calories: 316(per serving)
- Fat: 25.5g
- Protein: 15.2g
- Carbs: 4g

Broccoli Cheese Soup

Ingredients

- Ghee 1 tbsp.
- Onion 1 oz.
- Garlic cloves 2
- Heavy cream 4 oz.
- Vegetable broth 240 ml
- Water 240 ml
- Broccoli 6 oz.
- Cheddar cheese 4 oz.
- Salt and pepper to taste
- Paprika 1 tsp.
- Optional: coconut milk 2 tbsp.

Preparation Method

- Place a large soup pot over medium heat and add ghee. When ghee is hot add chopped onion, garlic and cook until translucent.
- Now, add cream, broth, water and boil for 15 minutes. Season with salt, pepper, and paprika.
- Meanwhile, cut broccoli into small florets and add to soup, reduce the heat to low and cook for 20 minutes.
- Once the broccoli is cooked, add shredded cheese and turn off the heat and serve in serving bowl.

- If desired, add 2 tbsp of coconut milk before serving and enjoy the soup

Nutritional Information

- Preparation Time: 45 minutes
- Total servings: 2
- Calories: 370 (per serving)
- Fat: 32g
- Protein: 14.4g
- Carbs: 7g

Salad Recipes

Spinach Infused Salad

Ingredients

- Spinach 2 oz.
- Hardboiled egg 1
- Bacon strips 2
- Chicken breast 2 oz.
- Grated mascarpone cheese 1 oz.
- Campari tomato 1 oz.
- Avocado 3 slices
- White vinegar 1 tsp.
- Ghee 2 tbsp.

Preparation Method

- At first, place a pan over medium heat and add 1 tbsp ghee. When ghee add bacon, chicken and cook until it turns to golden color.
- On the other hand, boil the spinach in water for 2 minutes and chop remaining ingredients in the desired size.
- In a mixing bowl, add all ingredients and mix well.

Nutritional Information

- Preparation Time: 20 minutes
- Total servings: 1
- Calories: 500 (per serving)

- Fat: 61g
- Protein: 41g
- Carbs: 5g

Fresh Herb Salad

Ingredients

- Mixed greens 1 oz.
- Mixed fresh herbs 1 oz. (Mint, Rosemary, Sage, Savory, Basil, Tarragon, Nasturtium)
- Roasted pine nuts 1 oz.
- Vinaigrette 1 ½ tbsp.
- Parmesan cheese 1 tbsp.
- Bacon slices 2
- Ghee 1 tbsp.
- Salt and pepper to taste

Preparation Method

- Cook bacon until crisp. Measure your greens, herbs and set in a container that can be shaken.
- Crumble bacon, then add the rest of the ingredients to the greens and shake the container with a lid.
- Add your seasonings and ghee for better taste and shake once again for proper dressing. Serve and enjoy the taste.

Nutritional Information

- Preparation Time: 10 minutes
- Total servings: 2
- Calories: 311 (per serving)

- Fat: 25.9g
- Protein: 8.9g
- Carbs: 2.9g

Cheesy Bean Salad

Ingredients

- Mixed beans 2 oz (cooked)
- Pine nuts 1 oz (roasted)
- Vinaigrette 4 tsp.
- Parmesan cheese 1 tbsp.
- Mozzarella cheese 1 oz.
- Bacon 2 slices
- Salt and pepper to taste

Preparation Method

- Cook bacon until crisp. Measure your beans and set in a container that can be shaken.
- Crumble bacon, then add the rest of the ingredients to the beans and shake the container with a lid.
- Add your seasonings for better taste and shake once again for proper dressing.
- Before serving, add mozzarella balls and enjoy the taste.

Nutritional Information

- Preparation Time: 10 minutes
- Serving per Recipe: 1
- Calories: 533 (per serving)
- Fat: 40.1g
- Protein: 17.9g
- Carbs: 5.8g

Heavy Greens

Ingredients

- Mixed greens 2 oz. (Spinach, Kale, Rapini, Collards)
- Roasted pine nuts 1 oz.
- Vinaigrette 4 tsp.
- Grated cheese 1 tbsp.
- Mozzarella cheese 1 oz. (small balls)
- Bacon 2 slices
- Salt and pepper to taste

Preparation Method

- Cook bacon until crisp. Measure your greens and set in a container that can be shaken.
- Crumble bacon, then add the rest of the ingredients to the greens and shake the container with a lid.
- Add your seasonings for better taste and shake once again for proper dressing.
- Before serving, add mozzarella balls and enjoy the taste.

Nutritional Information

- Preparation Time: 10 minutes
- Serving per Recipe: 1
- Calories: 553 (per serving)
- Fat: 41.6g
- Protein: 19.5g
- Carbs: 6.3g

Vegetable Salad

Ingredients

- Fresh tomato 1
- Vegetable mix 2 oz. (Cucumber, Carrot, Bell pepper, Beetroot)
- Fresh mozzarella cheese 6 oz.
- Turnip greens 1 tbsp.
- Fresh basil 1 ½ tbsp.
- Ghee 3 tbsp.
- Vinegar 1 tbsp.
- Fresh black pepper to taste
- Himalaya salt to taste

Preparation Method

- In a food processor, put chopped fresh basil, turnip leaves with ghee to make the paste.
- Slice tomato into 1/4" slices. You should be able to get at least 6 slices from the tomato and vegetables.
- Cut Mozzarella into slices. Assemble salad by layering tomato, mozzarella, and paste.
- Season with salt, pepper, and remaining ghee and enjoy the taste.

Nutritional Information

- Preparation Time: 12 minutes

- Serving per Recipe: 2
- Calories:433 (per serving)
- Fat: 40.5g
- Protein: 15.7g
- Carbs: 6.3g

Duck Parmesan Salad

Ingredients

- Duck breasts 14 oz.
- Bacon slices 4 oz.
- Romaine lettuce 1.76 lb.
- Salad Dressing 8 tbsp.
- Parmesan cheese flakes 4 oz.
- Salt and pepper to taste
- Anchovies 1 oz.

Preparation Method

- At first, preheat your oven to 375F and bake bacons until it becomes crispy approximately 15 minutes and keep aside.
- Now, make duck breast fry, by placing in oven to 430F, don't forget to season with salt and pepper. Cook for 15 minutes or until golden color and keep aside.
- Meanwhile, prepare dressing and other ingredients. Use a peeler to make the parmesan flakes and place the lettuce in a serving bowl and toss with the dressing.
- Now, slice the duck breasts into thin strips and place on top of the lettuce. Add the parmesan flakes and crisped up and crumbled bacon, anchovies and enjoy the taste.

Nutritional Information

- Preparation Time: 45 minutes

- Total servings: 4
- Calories: 707 (per serving)
- Fat: 60g
- Protein: 37g
- Carbs: 4g

Roasted Cheese Strawberry Salad

Ingredients

- Strawberries 5 oz.
- Goat cheese 5.3 oz.
- Pork rinds 1 oz.
- Pecans 2 oz.
- Fresh red and green lettuce 4.2 oz.
- Ghee 2 tbsp.
- Balsamic vinegar 1 tbsp.

Preparation Method

- At first, powder the pork rinds using a blender and keep aside.
- Now, cut each goat cheese in circular shape. Apply ghee and cover in powdered pork rinds. Place in freezer for 60 minutes to prevent the cheese from melting when grilled.
- Meanwhile, preheated your grill to 450F and cook cheese for just about 5 minutes.
- On other hand, wash strawberries, spray vinegar and place in oven at 450F for 10 minutes.
- Place washed lettuce in a serving bowl and add roasted pecans, drizzle the salad with ghee.
- Add the strawberry, grilled cheese to salad and enjoy your meal.

Nutritional Information

- Preparation Time: 75 minutes
- Total servings: 2
- Calories: 679 (per serving)
- Fat: 57g
- Protein: 28g
- Carbs: 9g

Green Leaf Salad

Ingredients

- Mixed green 56g
- Roasted macadamia nuts 30g
- Strawberry vinaigrette 20g
- Grated parmesan cheese 15g
- Bacon 2 slices
- Salt and pepper (as required)

Preparation Method

- Cook bacon until crispy. Measure your greens and put in a container that can be shaken.
- Crumble bacon, then add the rest of the ingredients to the greens and shake the container with a lid.
- Add your spices for better taste and slate once again for proper dressing. Serve and enjoy the taste.

Nutritional Information

- Preparation Time: 10 minutes
- Total servings: 1
- Calories: 478 (per serving)
- Fat: 39.2g
- Protein: 17.1g
- Carbs: 4.2g

Avocado Egg Salad

Ingredients

- Large hard boiled eggs 4
- Avocado 150g
- Mayonnaise 14g
- Yogurt 14g
- Chives 7g
- Red wine 10g
- Salt 2g
- Purified butter 20g
- Raw smashed pecans 28g
- Ground pepper to taste

Preparation Method

- Combine avocado, mayonnaise, yogurt, chives, vinegar, salt and pepper. Combine with smashed egg and adjust salt and pepper as needed. Sprinkle smashed pecans, purified butter and enjoy the taste.

Nutritional Information

- Preparation Time: 10 minutes
- Total servings: 6
- Calories: 210.4 (per serving)
- Fat: 18g
- Protein: 9.45g
- Carbs: 4.5g

Crab Salad

Ingredients
- Avocado 140g
- Crab meat 110g
- Chopped red onion 28g
- Fresh lime juice 20ml
- Chopped fresh coriander 14g
- Grape tomatoes 2
- Coconut oil 3gg
- Salt and fresh black pepper to taste
- Butter salad leaves 2
- Macadamia nuts 28g
- Tuna 28g

Preparation Method
- In a medium bowl, add onion, lemon juice, cilantro, tomato, olive oil, salt and fresh pepper. Add crab meat, tuna and sway lightly.
- Cut the avocado open, remove the pit and peel the skin or spoon out the avocado. Season with the remaining ingredients, fill the avocado halves evenly with crab salad and sprinkle smashed macadamia nuts. Serve immediately with butter leaves.

Nutritional Information

- Preparation Time: 15 minutes
- Total servings: 2
- Calories: 205.1 (per serving)
- Fat: 25g
- Protein: 14.75g
- Carbs:9g

Cheesy Salad Eggs

Ingredients

- Prosciutto 56g (4 slices)
- 5 cups of arugula 100g
- Parmesan cheese 25g
- Mascarpone cheese 28g
- Coconut oil 5ml
- Eggs 2
- Fresh black pepper to taste

Salad dressing:

- Chopped shallots 28g
- Olive oil 28g
- Vinegar 14g
- Dijon mustard 10g
- Raw honey 2g

Preparation Method

- Preheat oven to 375F. Place a large baking tray with parchment paper.
- Place the Prosciutto on the prepared baking tray and bake for 15 minutes or until lightly browned and crisp. Crumble into large pieces.

- In the meantime, beat the dressing ingredients in a large bowl. Divide on two plates and above with crushed prosciutto, parmesan and mascarpone cheese.
- To cook the eggs, heat a large non-stick pan over medium heat, spray with coconut oil and gently shake the eggs. Season with salt and cook until the white is set up and the egg yolk is still running, or longer if desired.
- Place the egg on each salad and serve with fresh pepper, if desired.

Nutritional Information

- Preparation Time: 20 minutes
- Total servings: 2
- Calories: 409 (per serving)
- Fat: 30.5g
- Protein: 19g
- Carbs:8g

Tofu Salad

Ingredients
- Tofu 420g
- Dark soy sauce 14g
- Sesame oil 14g
- Water 15g
- Mince garlic 8g
- Vinegar 10g
- Lemon juice 15g
- Chopped cilantro 14g

Preparation Method
- Cut the tofu and set aside and work on the marinating. Combine all ingredients such as soy sauce, sesame oil, water, garlic, vinegar and lemon.
- Mix the tofu and marinade mixture in a bowl and keep aside for 30 minutes. Preheat oven to 350F, place tofu on a baking tray covered with parchment paper and bake for 30 minutes.
- Once tofu is ready, sprinkle cilantro, lemon juice and enjoy the taste.

Nutritional Information
- Preparation Time: 65 minutes
- Total servings: 3

- Calories: 442.3 (per serving)
- Fat: 35g
- Protein: 22g
- Carbs: 5.5g

Snack Recipes

Broccoli Biscuits

Ingredients

- Almond flour 360g
- Raw broccoli florets 700g
- Cheddar cheese 125g
- Mascarpone cheese 112g
- Coconut oil 50g
- Large eggs 2
- Salt 5g
- Garlic powder 5g
- Baking soda 2g
- Pepper 5g
- Apple cider 3g

Preparation Method

- Heat your oven to 375F, blend broccoli flowers until it is finely chopped.
- In a large bowl, mix almond flour, salt, peppers, garlic powder, baking soda. Mix it well, add eggs and coconut oil. Mix until a dough forms.
- Add your broccoli to the mixture. Combine everything with your hands. Grate cheddar and mascarpone. Cheese's to the dough. Mix everything with the hands until the cheese is evenly distributed.

- Place your non-stick silpat on a cookie sheet, so that they do not stick as they boil. Form pies from the dough. Bake like biscuits for 15 minutes or until they begin to flatten.
- Turn it and continue baking for about 5 minutes then, turn your oven to roast and brew the biscuits for 3 minutes.
- Let it cool for 2 minutes and enjoy the taste.

Nutritional Information

- Preparation Time: 30 minutes
- Total servings: 12
- Calories: 206.3 (per serving)
- Fat: 18.6g
- Protein: 7.2g
- Carbs: 2.5g

Coconut Fat Bombs

Ingredients
- Coconut oil 100g
- Heavy whipped cream 115g
- Fresh cheese 110g
- Pineapple extract 5g
- Stevia 10 drops
- Protein powder 28g

Preparation Method
- At first, mix coconut oil, heavy cream and fresh cheese. Using a mixer, mix all the ingredients together or place in microwave oven for 30 seconds to 1 minute to soften them.
- Add orange vanilla extract and liquid stevia to the mixture and mix with a spoon.
- Distribute the mixture into a silicone tray and freeze for 3 hours.

Nutritional Information
- Preparation Time: 15 minutes
- Total servings: 10
- Calories: 186 (per serving)
- Fat: 20g
- Protein: 2.8g
- Carbs: 0.7g

Crunchy Crackers

Ingredients

- Almond flour 300g
- Purified butter 42g
- Black pepper 2g
- Salt 2g
- Baking soda 2g
- Dried basil 2g
- Cayenne pepper 1g
- Garlic clove 1
- Basil 28g

Preparation Method

- Preheat oven to 325F. Place a cookie sheet with parchment paper. In a medium bowl, mix almond flour, pepper, salt and baking powder.
- Add basil, cayenne and garlic and stir until uniformly combined. Next, add to the pesto and snowbake until the dough forms into coarse crumbs. Cut the butter into the cracker mixture with a fork until the dough forms a ball.
- Transfer the dough to the prepared cookie sheet and spread the dough thinly until it is about 1 mm thick. Make sure the thickness is the same, so that the biscuits evenly bake.

- Place the pan in the pre-heated oven and bake for 15 minutes to light golden brown color. After baking, remove from the oven and cut into biscuits of the desired size.

Nutritional Information

- Preparation Time: 25 minutes
- Total servings: 6
- Calories:210 (per serving)
- Fat: 20g
- Protein: 5g
- Carbs: 3g

Pumpkin Bars

Ingredients

- Coconut butter 260g
- Pumpkin purees 225g
- Ground cinnamon 4g
- Peanuts 3g
- Cashew butter 100g
- Protein powder 50g
- Coconut oil 14g

Preparation Method

- Hold aside 8x8 inch square baking tray with aluminum foil. In the large bowl, add melted coconut butter, cashew butter, pumpkin spices, spices, protein powder and mix well.
- Add coconut oil and combine well without lumps. Pour the mixture into the already prepared pan and spread evenly.
- Cover with wax paper and evenly put into the pan. Remove wax paper and place the mixture in the refrigerator for 3 hours.
- Use a sharp knife to cut into 25 equal squares and enjoy the delicious taste.

Nutritional Information

- Preparation Time: 15 minutes
- Total servings: 25

- Calories: 150 (per serving)
- Fat: 11.28g
- Protein: 4.76g
- Carbs: 2.2g

Coconut Cashew Bar

Ingredients

- Almond flour 140g
- Butter 55g
- Maple syrup 30g
- Cinnamon 4g
- Salt to taste
- Cashew nuts 75g
- Protein powder 50g
- Shredded coconut 15g

Preparation Method

- Combine almond flour and melted butter in a large bowl. Add cinnamon, salt and maple syrup, protein powder and mix well.
- Add crushed coconut and mix again. Add chopped cashews and mix everything evenly.
- Pour parchment paper into a casserole dish and spread the dough in a flat layer. Sprinkle crushed coconut and cinnamon up for beautiful crispy flavor.
- Place them in a refrigerator and cool for 3 hours (night will give the best result). Cut into bars and enjoy the taste.

Nutritional Information

- Preparation Time:15 minutes

- Total servings: 8
- Calories: 211.5 (per serving)
- Fat: 17g
- Protein: 8.2g
- Carbs: 4.1g

Fish Stuffed Taco

Ingredients

- Ghee 2 tbsp.
- Red onion 2 oz.
- Fresh jalapeno 0.5 oz.
- Garlic clove 1
- Mascarpone cheese 2 oz.
- Heavy cream 1 oz.
- Adobo sauce 2 oz.
- Mayonnaise 1 tbsp.
- Haddock fillets 0.5 lb.
- Low carb tortillas 2

Preparation Method

- Place a pan over a medium heat and add ghee, when ghee is hot, add diced onion. Cook for 5 minutes or until translucent.
- Add the chopped jalapeno, garlic and stir for another 2 minutes.
- Add adobo sauce to the pan and stir for another minute. Now, add fish fillets to the pan and mix well and cook for 10 minutes until the fish is fully cooked then turn off the heat and add cheese, cream,
- Meanwhile, warm the tortillas using 1 tbsp ghee over it and stuff the fish and enjoy the taste,

Nutritional Information

- Preparation Time: 20 minutes
- Total servings: 2
- Calories: 481 (per serving)
- Fat: 40g
- Protein: 25.4g
- Carbs: 8.2g

Double Meat Fries

Ingredients

- Almond Meal 1 1/3 cup
- Large eggs 2
- Pork sausages 2
- Beef sausages 2
- Olive oil 150g (for frying)
- Heavy cream 1 oz.
- Baking powder 1 tsp.
- Allspice 1 tsp.
- Salt ½ tsp.
- Cayenne Pepper ½ tsp.

Preparation Method

- In a mixing bowl, add almond flour, allspice and mix all the dry ingredients well so they are completely distributed,
- Add your eggs, baking powder, heavy cream to the batter and mix everything well until a nice thick batter is formed,
- In a saucepan, heat olive oil to 400F. Cut each sausage into 2 piece and mix half pork and half beef sausage into single sausage; dip mixed sausages in the batter before you fry them. Make sure they're fully coated,
- Drop your sausage into the oil 1 at a time. Let it cook for 3 minutes on one side, then flip it and cook for about 2 minutes on the other side,

- Remove your sausages from the pan and let it dry on some paper towels. Dish out with some hot sauces and enjoy the taste.

Nutritional Information

- Preparation Time: 10 minutes
- Serving per Recipe: 4
- Calories:380.2 (per serving)
- Fat: 36.1g
- Protein: 17.2g
- Carbs: 4.9g

Grilled Mushroom

Ingredients

- Mushroom 12 oz.
- Olive oil 2 tbsp.
- Balsamic vinegar 2 tbsp.
- Rosemary 1/2 tsp.
- Tarragon 1/2 tsp.
- Basil 1/2 tsp.
- Thyme 1/2 tsp.
- Sea salt to taste

Preparation Method

- At first, preheat your grill. Whisk olive oil, balsamic vinegar, and herbs together,
- Now, slice mushroom about 1/2" thick and brush with already whisked herb mixture onto both sides of your mushroom,
- Lay the slices down on your preheated grill and cook for about 3 minutes on both sides,
- Before serving sprinkle sea salt and enjoy the taste,

Nutritional Information

- Preparation Time: 15 minutes
- Total servings: 4

- Calories: 84 (per serving)
- Fat:7 g
- Protein: 3.3g
- Carbs: 2g

Grilled Cheese Kale

Ingredients
- Kale leaves 30
- Ghee 1 tbsp.
- Grape wine 1 tbsp.
- Fresh thyme leaves 1 tsp.
- Fresh dill 1 tsp.
- Garlic cloves 2
- Macadamia nuts 1 oz.
- Pumpkin seeds 1 oz.
- Parmesan cheese 1 oz

Preparation Method
- At first, preheat the oven to 400F. I like 10 kale leaves per person, depending on their size. Cut both ends and peel back the first or second layer of leaves and discard. Leave the kale in a pan with boiling salt water for 2 minutes.
- Drain well and place in a bowl of ghee, grape wine, chopped thyme leaves, dill and garlic. Spread the kale in a layer in a baking tray, sprinkle nuts, pumpkin seeds and cheese. Bake for 10 minutes until it is caramelized.

Nutritional Information
- Preparation Time: 15 minutes

- Total servings: 3
- Calories: 151 (10 kale leaves per serving)
- Fat: 15.5g
- Protein: 6.5g
- Carbs: 3.3g

Dessert Recipes

Frozen Pumpkin Cups

Ingredients
- Heavy cream 8.2 oz.
- Pumpkin pie spice 1 tsp.
- Egg yolks 2
- Erythritol 2 tbsp.
- Pumpkins puree 2 tbsp.
- Powdered sugar for topping

Preparation Method
- At first, preheat your oven to 300F. Place saucepan over medium heat and add heavy cream then add pumpkin pie spice,
- After 5 minutes or until you see bubbles turn off the heat and keep aside, In a small bowl, add egg yolks and whisk until it changes color to light yellow.
- Now add egg mixture to cream mixture and whisking continuously then add pumpkin puree, erythritol. Mix well,
- Put this batter in a 2 muffin cup and bake in a preheated oven for 30 minutes or until top turns to light brown color then place in refrigerator for at least 4 hours.
- Before serving sprinkle powdered sugar and enjoy the taste.

Nutritional Information
- Preparation Time: 50 minutes

- Total servings: 2
- Calories: 460 (per serving)
- Fat: 49g
- Protein: 15g
- Carbs: 5g

Ricotta Strawberries

Ingredients
- Large eggs 2
- Coconut flour 2 tbsp.
- Ricotta cheese 3.5 oz.
- Mascarpone cheese 1 oz.
- Vanilla beans extract ½ tsp.
- Ghee 1 tbsp.
- Cream of tartar ½ tsp.
- Baking soda ¼ tsp.
- Fresh strawberries 2.5 oz.
- Stevia 10 drops

Preparation Method
- At first, preheat your oven to 350F. In a separate bowl add egg yolks, vanilla extract, ricotta cheese, mascarpone and stevia.
- Other side, beat egg whites with baking soda and cream of tartar untill they become thick and form soft peaks.
- Now add egg whites mixture to egg yolk mixture and very gently fold in and slowly add the coconut flour.
- Place the sliced strawberries onto a baking dish lined with parchment paper and greased with ghee.
- Top with the pancake mixture and add more strawberries on top. Spray with ghee and place in preheated oven.

- Set timer to 15 minutes until slightly browned and serve warm.

Nutritional Information

- Preparation Time: 25 minutes
- Total servings: 2
- Calories: 342 (per serving)
- Fat: 26.5g
- Protein: 15g
- Carbs: 6g

Cream Pots

Ingredients
- Heavy cream 260g
- Powdered erythritol 1 oz.
- Liquid stevia ½ tsp.
- Pinch of salt
- Egg yolks 4
- Water 75g
- Maple syrup 1 tbsp.
- Vanilla extracts ½ tsp.
- Maples extract 2 tsp.

Preparation Method
- Preheat the oven to 300F and whisk egg yolks finely.
- Mix water with erythritol in small pan and start boiling on low heat. After 1 minute, add maple syrup and keep aside.
- In another medium bowl, mix cream, stevia, salt, extracts and start boiling on low heat and add water syrup (first bowl) into batter and add whisk egg yolk.
- Mix well until it looks smooth and soft. Add to small cups and keep in oven for 10-15 minutes or until it looks like the pudding texture and sprinkle with cinnamon for flavor and enjoy the taste

Nutritional Information

- Preparation Time: 20 minutes
- Serving per Recipe: 4
- Calories: 359 (per serving)
- Fat: 34.9g
- Protein: 2.8g
- Carbohydrates: 3g

Coffee Cake

Ingredients

Base:

- Eggs 6
- Cream cheese 150g
- Erythritol 50g
- Liquid stevia 1 oz.
- Optional: protein powder 1 oz.
- Vanilla extract 8g
- Cream of tartar 1 oz.

Filling:

- Almond flour 210g
- Cinnamon 1 tbsp.
- Butter 115g
- Maple syrup 1 oz.
- Erythritol 1 oz.
-

Preparation Method

- Preheat the oven to 325F. In large bowl, add egg, erythritol and liquid stevia and mix well using hand mixer.
- Add cream cheese, protein powder and mix well until a thick batter forms. Mix egg into the tartar cream and pour the batter into a round cake pan.

- Mix together all filling ingredients and make dough and take half and rip off the little pieces on top the cake and push down in cake batter.
- Bake for 20 minutes and top with cinnamon filling and bake for another 20 minutes until a toothpick comes out clean.
- Cool it for 20 minutes and slice into 8 pieces and enjoy the taste.

Nutritional Information

- Preparation Time: 70 minutes
- Serving per Recipe: 8
- Calories: 257 (per serving)
- Fat: 26.7g
- Protein: 12.8g
- Carbohydrates: 3.8g

Coco filled Brownies

Ingredients

- Cocoa powder 2 cups
- Almond flour ½ cup
- Sweetener 1 ½ tbsp.
- Coconut oil 2 fl oz.
- Maple syrup 1oz
- Large eggs 2
- Caramel 2 tsp.
- Baking powder ½ tsp.
- Salt to taste

Preparation Method

- At first, preheat oven to 350F. In the meantime, add sweetener, coconut oil, maple syrup, eggs, and caramel in a bowl.
- In the separate bowl, combine all the cocoa powder, almond flour, baking powder and salt. Mix bowl1 and bowl2 with hand mixer.
- Put the dough into a 10x8 baking pan and bake for 25 minutes. Let the brownies cool for 5 minutes and cut them into 8 equal parts and enjoy the taste.

Nutritional Information

- Preparation Time: 35 minutes

- Total servings: 8
- Calories: 263 (per serving)
- Fat: 24.1g
- Protein: 7.9g
- Carbs: 3.8g

Hot Donuts

Ingredients

- Almond flour 100g
- Flaxseed flour 35g
- Sweetener 30g
- Pineapple extract 4g
- Baking powder 4g
- Eggs 2
- Coconut oil 24g
- Coconut milk 50g
- Chocolate 10g
- Berry extracts 8g
- Food color 10 drops
- Salt to taste

Preparation Method

- Combine almond flour, flaxseed flour, sweetener, baking soda and a pinch of salt, mix well.
- Combine eggs, pineapple extract, coconut oil, coconut milk and make smooth dough. Add chocolate to the dough, berry extract and food color.
- Stir well until the dough is even. Connect the donut maker and place the dough into the hot donut maker and close for 5 minutes before you turn.

- Turn around and cook for 2 minutes and enjoy the hot donuts.

Nutritional Information

- Preparation Time: 30 minutes
- Total servings: 12
- Calories: 107 (per serving)
- Fat: 9g
- Protein: 3g
- Carbs: 1.2g

Pumpkin Pie

Ingredients
- Butter 115g
- Erythritol 30 g
- Egg 1
- Stevia 15 drops
- Cinnamon 4g
- Pumpkin purees 40g
- Vanilla extract 4g
- Pumpkin spice 3g
- Almond flour 35g
- Coconut flour 28g
- Chopped Pecans 28g
- Pumpkin seeds 28g
- Protein powder 28g

Preparation Method
- Preheat the oven to 375F and combine your butter and erythritol with the blender.
- Add the egg, cinnamon, stevia, pumpkin puree, pumpkin cake spice and maple extract, mix well. Finally, add the almond flour, protein powder and the coconut powder and mix well.

- On brownie pan, spray coconut oil and spread dough in a level layer. Chop pecans, pumpkin seeds and sprinkle them over the surface of the blondies.
- Bake for 20-25 minutes or until top layer becomes slightly brown. Enjoy with a glass of coffee or tea.

Nutritional Information

- Preparation Time: 30 minutes
- Total servings: 12
- Calories: 133.58 (per serving)
- Fat: 13.62g
- Protein: 4.7g
- Carbs: 1.7g

Creamy Mousse

Ingredients

Cream cheese mixture:

- Cream cheese 225g
- Sour cream 42g
- Purified butter 25g
- Vanilla extract 8g
- Granulated erythritol powder 70g
- Cocoa powder 25g
- Instant coffee powder 15g

Whipped cream mixture:

- Heavy whipping cream 150g
- Erythritol powder 8g
- Pineapple extract 2g

Garnish:

- Smashed pumpkin seeds 28g

Preparation Method

- At first, take a medium bowl; beat sour cream, ghee, cream cheese until smooth using electric mixer.
- Now, add erythritol, cocoa powder, vanilla extract, coffee powder and blend until it mixed well. Set aside.

- In another separate bowl, add whipping cream, erythritol, vanilla extract and beat until stiff peaks form.
- Mix whipped cream mixture into the cream cheese mixture until it incorporated well and transfer the final mixture into serving cups.
- Sprinkle smashed pumpkin seeds and refrigerate until serving (for better taste and result refrigerate for 150 minutes).

Nutritional Information

- Preparation Time: 25 minutes
- Total servings: 4
- Calories: 464.4
- Fat: 46.5g
- Protein: 7.5g
- Carbs: 5.25g

Mocha Coconut Cake

Ingredients

- Coconut flour 2 tbsp.
- Large egg 1
- Cocoa powder 1 tbsp.
- Mocha powder 1 tbsp.
- Baking powder 1 tsp.
- Vanilla sugar 1 tsp.
- Stevia 2 tbsp.
- Ghee 1 tbsp.
- Cream 2 tbsp.
- Optional: top with almond flakes

Preparation Method

- At first, place all your dry ingredients in a mug and combine well.
- Add the egg, ghee, stevia and mix well using a fork. Place in microwave on high for 90 seconds.
- Before serving, add cream and enjoy the taste.

Nutritional Information

- Preparation Time: 5 minutes
- Total servings: 1
- Calories:332 (per serving)

- Fat: 30.6g
- Protein: 11.2g
- Carbs: 5.2g

White Raspberry Ice Cream

Ingredients

- Heavy cream 8.2 oz.
- Erythritol 2 oz
- Raspberries 6 oz.
- Protein powder 2 oz.
- Large egg yolks 3
- Vanilla extracts 1/2 tsp.
- Xanthan Gum 1/8 tsp.
- Vodka 1 tbsp.

Preparation Method

- Place a pan over simmer and add heavy cream, erythritol, don't boil it just wait until erythritol is dissolved gently.
- Meanwhile, add egg yolks in mixing bowl and beat using hand mixer until they've doubled in size.
- Now, add hot cream mixture gently into the egg mixture and mix. Add vanilla extract, protein powder, xanthan gum and mix well.
- If desired, add vodka and place your bowl in the freezer for 2 hours minimum, don't forget stir occasionally.
- Meanwhile, put raspberries in a mixer (it should be little chunky). When the ice cream looks bit thicker, it's right time to add the chunky raspberries and mix gently, but don't over mix.

- Let this ice cream chill for another 4 hours or overnight before it tastes it.

Nutritional Information

- Preparation Time: 330 minutes
- Total servings: 6
- Calories: 211 (per serving)
- Fat: 17g
- Protein: 8g
- Carbs: 2.3g

Lime Cream Cake

Ingredients

Base

- Eggs 3
- Egg whites 3
- Butter 4 oz.
- Heavy whipping cream 8 oz.
- Lime zest 1 tsp.
- Almond flour 7 oz.
- Coconut flour 1.5 oz.
- Protein powder 1 oz.
- Erythritol 2 oz.
- Baking soda 1/2 tsp.
- Cream of tartar 1 tsp.
- Salt 1/4 tsp.

Filling

- Egg yolks 3
- Fresh lime juice 4 fl oz.
- Lime zest 1 tbsp.
- Condensed Milk 8.5 oz.
- Ghee 2 oz.

Topping

- Heavy whipping cream 8 fl oz.
- Fresh lime zest 1 tsp.

Preparation Method

- At first, preheat your oven to 325F. We will start preparing cake base, take 8 x 8-inch pan with parchment paper.
- In a large bowl, mix all base ingredients and whisk using hand mixer until it mixed well.
- Place in preheated oven and bake for 30 minutes or until the top is lightly golden and keep aside. Meanwhile, in a bowl, mix all filling ingredients until it becomes thick curd paste.
- Using fork make holes all over the cake base. Apply curd paste all over the cake base until covered and the holes are filled. Place in the fridge for 60 minutes.
- After 60 minutes, spread cream all over the cake and sprinkle with freshly grated lime zest. Again put in fridge for 60 minutes and enjoy the taste.

Nutritional Information

- Preparation Time: 200 minutes
- Total servings: 12
- Calories: 447 (per serving)
- Fat: 43.2g
- Protein: 10.5g
- Carbs: 5.5g

Carrot Loaves

Ingredients

- Carrots 13.8 oz.
- Flax Meal 2.1 oz.
- Pumpkin seeds 1.8 oz.
- Sunflower seeds 1.4 oz
- Ghee 3 tbsp.
- Eggs 2
- Fresh thyme 1 tbsp.
- Salt to taste
- Sesame oil 1 tbsp.

Preparation Method

- At first, preheat the oven to 375F and grease your baking tray (8 x 4) to avoid sticking.
- Now, peel and remove skin and tops of the carrots, chop into chunks and blitz in a food processor until it comes to rice consistency.
- In a small bowl, whisk eggs with a fork and mix the blitzed carrots, flaxseed meal, pumpkin seeds, sunflower seeds, ghee, salt and fresh thyme together.
- Put this mixture into the already greased baking tray and bake in preheated oven for about 40 minutes.
- Let it cool for 10 minutes and before you serve drizzle with sesame oil and fresh thyme.

Nutritional Information

- Preparation Time: 50 minutes
- Total servings: 4
- Calories: 405 (per serving)
- Fat: 36.7g
- Protein: 13g
- Carbs: 8g

Marjoram Cake

Ingredients

Base:

- Large eggs 6
- Cream cheese 6 oz.
- Erythritol 1 ½ oz.
- Protein powder 1 oz.
- Vanillas extract 2 tsp.
- Cream of tartar 1 tsp.
- Ghee 2 tbsp.

Filling:

- Almond flour 1 cup
- Marjoram 2 tsp.
- Cinnamon 1 tsp.
- Ghee 3 oz.
- Maple syrup 1 ½ oz.
- Erythritol 1 ½ oz.

Preparation Method

- At first, preheat your oven to 325F.
- In a bowl, mix all base ingredients and mix together well until a thick batter forms and stiff peaks form.

- Mix together all of the filling ingredients in a bowl. Now, add base mixture in cake pan and bake for 20 minutes and then top with filling mixture.
- Bake for another 20 minutes until a toothpick comes out clean. Let cool for 20 minutes before removing from the cake pan to enjoy the taste.

Nutritional Information

- Preparation Time: 50 minutes
- Serving per Recipe: 8
- Calories: 257 (per serving)
- Fat: 36.5g
- Protein: 13.3g
- Carbohydrates: 5.1g

Cheese Filled Buns

Ingredients

- Eggs 2
- Almond flour 2 tablespoons
- Husk powder 1 tablespoon
- Baking powder 1/2 teaspoon
- Ghee/purified butter 2 tablespoons
- Cheddar cheese 2 ounces (filling)
- Mascarpone 1 ounce (filling)

Preparation Method

- At first, we will make buns. In a mixing bowl, add ghee/purified butter, almond flour, husk, baking powder, eggs and mix together until it forms a thick dough.
- Pour the dough into a square bowl and place in microwave for about 90 seconds and cut in half using a bread knife.
- Now, add cheddar, mascarpone cheeses in between the buns. Heat butter in pan and add bun and allow cooking for 2 minutes each or until it looks crispy outside and enjoying the tasty sandwich.

Nutritional Information

- Preparation Time: 5 minutes
- Total servings: 1
- Calories: 630 (per serving)
- Fat: 69.81g

- Protein:16.1 g
- Carbs: 3.8g

Raspberry Pudding

Ingredients

- Coconut flour 1.2 ounce
- Raspberry 1.5 ounce
- Baking powder 1/4 teaspoon
- Egg yolks 5
- Protein powder 2 teaspoons
- Coconut oil 2 tablespoons
- Purified butter 2 tablespoons
- Sour cream 2 tablespoons
- Lemon juice 2 teaspoons
- Lemon zest 2 teaspoons
- Erythritol 2 tablespoons
- Stevia 10 drops

Preparation Method

- At first, preheat your oven to 350F. In separate bowl, add egg yolks, coconut flour, baking powder, coconut oil, purified butter, mix well and set aside for 5 minutes.
- Now, add erythritol, stevia, sour cream, lemon juice, zest, mix well until no lumps are found.
- Add batter to 2 ramekins or muffin cups and lightly push the raspberries with your finger into batter and also cut berries into small pieces and sprinkle over the batter.

- Place in preheated oven and bake for 25 minutes at 350F, let it cool for 5 minutes. If desired, add heavy whipping cream over the top and enjoy the taste.

Nutritional Information

- Preparation Time: 30 minutes
- Total servings: 2
- Calories: 507.5 (per serving)
- Fat: 43.5g
- Protein: 17.6g
- Carbs: 6g

Macadamia Custard

Ingredients

- Coconut milk 220ml
- Eggs 4
- Heavy cream 80g
- Macadamia nut butter 60g
- Erythritol 35g
- Liquid stevia 4g
- Vanilla extract 4g

Preparation Method

- Preheat the oven to 325F. In a bowl, add coconut milk, heavy cream, vanilla extract, eggs and start whisking (slowly).
- Add stevia and macadamia butter and continue stirring until it mixed evenly.
- Fill a small baking pan with about 1 inch of water and place your baking cups in water and add your custard mixture.
- Bake it for 40-45 minutes and cool it for 20 minutes. Enjoy the delicious taste

Nutritional Information

- Preparation Time: 75 minutes
- Serving per Recipe: 13

- Calories: 275 (per serving)
- Fat: 26.2g
- Protein: 6.2g
- Carbohydrates: 2.5g

Smoothie Recipes

Tropical Smoothie

Ingredients

- Ice cubes 7
- Coconut milk 185g
- Sour cream 60g
- Flaxseed meal 1 oz.
- Coconut oil 1 tbsp.
- Liquid stevia 20 drops
- Blueberries extract ½ tsp.

Preparation Method

- In blender, place all ingredients and blend on medium speed or until smooth.
- Pour into serving glass and enjoy the taste.

Nutritional Information

- Preparation Time: 5 minutes
- Serving per Recipe: 1
- Calories:352 (per serving)
- Fat: 31g
- Protein: 5g
- Carbohydrates: 3g

Cinnamon Smoothies

Ingredients
- Almond milk 245g
- Protein powder 1 oz.
- Cinnamon 1 tsp.
- Vanilla extract 3 drops
- Sweetener 20g
- Flax meal 1 tsp.
- Ice 140g

Preparation Method
- In blender, place all ingredients and blend on medium speed or until smooth.
- Pour into serving glass and enjoy the taste.

Nutritional Information
- Preparation Time: 5 minutes
- Serving per Recipe: 1
- Calories:145 (per serving)
- Fat: 3.25g
- Protein: 26.5g
- Carbohydrates: 0.6g

Protein Mint Smoothie

Ingredients

- Avocado ½ piece
- Spinach 225g
- Whey protein powder 1 oz.
- Almond milk 122g
- Stevia 10 drops
- Peppermint extract 3 drops
- Ice 140g

Preparation Method

- In blender, place all ingredients and blend on medium speed or until smooth.
- Pour into serving glass and enjoy the taste.

Nutritional Information

- Preparation Time: 5 minutes
- Serving per Recipe: 1
- Calories:225 (per serving)
- Fat: 13.3g
- Protein: 20.7g
- Carbohydrates: 9.4g

Yogurt Smoothie

Ingredients

- Greek Yogurt 70g
- Frozen blueberries 45g
- Almond milk 80g
- Spinach 225g
- Vanilla protein powder 28g
- Ice 45g

Preparation Method

- In blender, place all ingredients and blend on medium speed or until smooth.
- Pour into serving glass and enjoy the taste.

Nutritional Information

- Preparation Time: 5 minutes
- Serving per Recipe: 1
- Calories:290 (per serving)
- Fat: 13.5g
- Protein: 9g
- Carbohydrates: 4g

Mocha Smoothie

Ingredients

- Coconut milk 490g
- Instant coffee 2 teaspoons
- Cocoa powder 3g
- Coconut extract 1 drop
- Packet stevia 100g

Preparation Method

- In blender, place all ingredients and blend on medium speed or until smooth.
- Pour into serving glass and enjoy the taste.

Nutritional Information

- Preparation Time: 5 minutes
- Serving per Recipe: 1
- Calories:120 (per serving)
- Fat: 10g
- Protein: 2g
- Carbohydrates: 2g

Berry Smoothie

Ingredients

- Flax seed meal 1 oz.
- Chia seeds 1 tbsp.
- Coconut milk 450ml
- Liquid stevia 10 drops
- Blueberries 85g
- Bananas extract 1 tsp.
- Ice cubes 7

Preparation Method

- Blend the coconut milk with 7 ice cubes, banana extract, stevia.
- Add blueberries, flax meal, chia seed and blend until ingredients are fully incorporated.
- Measure out into serving and enjoy the taste.

Nutritional Information

- Preparation Time: 10 minutes
- Serving per Recipe: 2
- Calories: 264 (per serving)
- Fat: 25g
- Protein: 4g
- Carbohydrates: 3g

Frozen Strawberry Smoothie

Ingredients

- Frozen strawberries 150g
- Coconut milk 1 cup
- Almond butter 1 oz.
- Stevia 10 drops

Preparation Method

- Add all ingredients into the blender and blend until smooth.
- Pour into glass and enjoy the taste.

Nutritional Information

- Preparation Time: 10 minutes
- Serving per Recipe: 2
- Calories: 52 (per serving)
- Fat: 2.3g
- Protein: 0.3g
- Carbohydrates: 1.6g

Avocado Rasp Smoothie

Ingredients

- Peeled avocado 1
- Water 1 cup
- Lemon juice 4 tsp.
- Stevia 10 drops
- Frozen raspberries 85g

Preparation Method

- Add all ingredients into the blender and blend until smooth.
- Pour into two glasses and enjoy the taste with straw.

Nutritional Information

- Preparation Time: 10 minutes
- Serving per Recipe: 2
- Calories: 227 (330ml per serving)
- Fat: 20g
- Protein: 2.5g
- Carbohydrates: 12g

Blackberry Smoothie

Ingredients

- Coconut milk 1 cup
- Blackberries 650g
- Cocoa powder 1 ½ tbsp.
- Ice cubes 7
- Stevia 12 drops

Preparation Method

- Add all ingredients into the blender and blend until smooth.
- Pour into glass and enjoy the taste with straw.

Nutritional Information

- Preparation Time: 5 minutes
- Serving per Recipe: 1
- Calories: 338
- Fat: 34g
- Protein: 1g
- Carbohydrates: 4g

Cream Smoothie

Ingredients

- Heavy whipping cream 80g
- Almond milk 120ml
- Frozen mixed berries 75g
- Extra virgin coconut oil 2 tsp.
- Ice cubes 5
- Stevia 3 drops
- Vanilla extract ½ tsp.

Preparation Method

- Add all ingredients into the blender and blend until smooth.
- Pour into glass and enjoy the taste with straw.

Nutritional Information

- Preparation Time: 10 minutes
- Serving per Recipe: 1
- Calories: 400
- Fat: 41g
- Protein: 4g
- Carbohydrates: 7g

Free Keto Diet Simplified Book

Hey! Want a free book? Check out my website and get a FREE copy of **Keto Diet Simplified**.

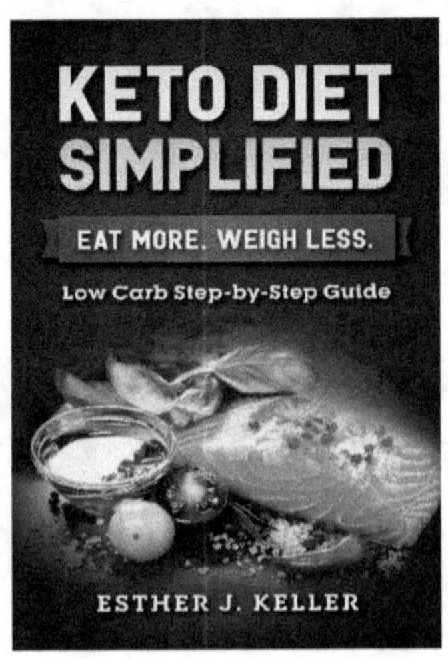

Simply go to: www.EstherFitness.com

No strings attached. Promise.

Yours,

Leave a Review

If you found this short book was helpful at all or provided even a small insight that you took away, would you consider helping other people find this book by leaving this book an honest review? That'd mean a lot!

About the Author

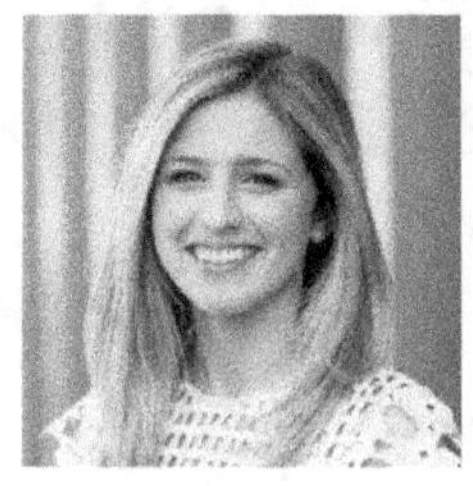 Esther Keller is a journalist by day and a runner by night. She loves long runs with her dog Russell and bike rides on chilly nights. She studied journalism at the University of Michigan and moved to Brooklyn upon graduating where she works as a fitness instructor. She loves reading, eating, exercising, hiking, sleeping and watching the Power Puff girls and New Girl.

Copyright

© 2017 Esther J. Keller

First Edition

Ketogenic Diet

The Complete Guide to Healthy Weight Loss

Step by Step Guide + 55 recipes + 14-Day Meal Plan